SECRETS OF STRENGTH AND DEVELOPMENT

(ORIGINAL VERSION, RESTORED)

BY BOB HOFFMAN

"The world's leading physical director" - Editor in Chief of
Strength and Health Magazine

Originally Published in 1940

PUBLISHED BY O'Faolain Patriot LLC, Copyright 2011

info@PhysicalCultureBooks.com

ISBN-13: 978-1468066203

ISBN-10: 146806620X

Published in the United States of America

To Order More Copies Visit: Physical Culture Books.com

TABLE OF CONTENTS

I. MEN SHOULD BE STRONG   p.5

II. CAN STRENGTH BE ACQUIRED?   p.24

III. INHERITED PHYSICAL STRENGTH   p.45

IV. BONE SIZE IN REGARD TO STRENGTH   p.67

V. TENDON AND LIGAMENT STRENGTH   p.93

VI. IMPORTANCE OF SIZE AND WEIGHT   p.113

VII. DEVELOPMENT OF MUSCLE AS A MEANS TO STRENGTH AND PERFECT PROPORTIONS   p.127

VIII. STRENGTH THROUGH SYMMETRICAL DEVELOPMENT   p.141

IX. STRENGTH AND DEVELOPMENT AS A RESULT OF NATURAL ADVANTAGES   p.159

X. STRENGTH THROUGH QUALITY OF MUSCLE   p.175

XI. ALL-AROUND DEVELOPMENT   p.190

XII. THE RESULT OF SUPERIOR TRAINING METHODS   p.202

XIII. ADDITIONAL SUCCESSFUL TRAINING PRINCIPLES   p.216

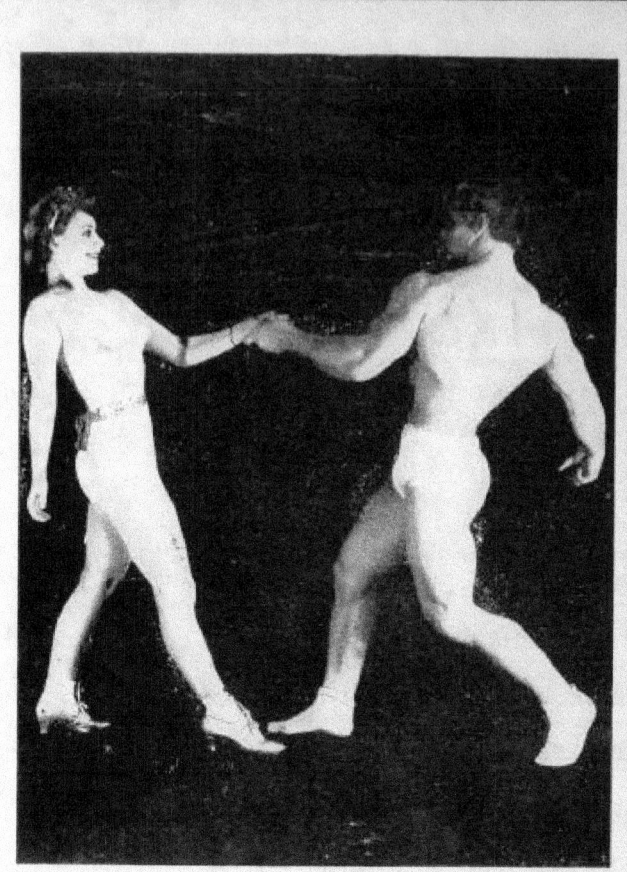

Masculine and feminine perfection. Gracie Bard and John Grimek. Gracie is a professional dancer who improved her physique by moderate training with weights and cables. She is 5' 2" in height, and weighs 114 pounds. Has chinned herself 15 repetitions and two hand pressed 100 pounds.

CHAPTER ONE
Men Should Be Strong

Breathes there a man with soul so dead,
Who never to himself hath said,
I want to be strong and well developed.

Few men grow to manhood without at some time during their early life passing through a period when their greatest desire is to be a strong man. They may know some man who is especially strong and wish to be like him. They may have visited the circus or the theatre and seen a powerful man who is their ideal. For at least a period they are filled with a desire to emulate the deeds of their temporary hero.

There is no subject quite as fascinating to most young men as the subject of strength and development. The principal source of their conversation may be the deeds of their favorite athletic hero: a baseball player such as Babe Ruth or Joe DiMaggio; a football player like Biggie Goldberg, the great Pittsburgh halfback, or Ernie Nevers, the Pacific Coast fullback star of a few years ago; it may be George O'Brien of the movies, or one of the series of movie Tarzans—Buster Crabbe, Johnny Weismuller, or Glen Morris. But the strength of the man is what they really admire, for it was strength and development more than any other physical or mental characteristic which made these men stars of the playing field or the movies.

If you wish to prove my assertion that strength is more admired or talked about than any other subject among young fellows, start a discussion among your friends about strong men. Just tell your friends that a relative of yours, or some other friend or acquaintance, is certainly the strongest fellow in town, and then listen to the outbursts of rhetoric as each one tells of someone he knows who is the strongest man in town, or in the state, or even in the world.

You will be besieged with questions as to what your friend can do, how strong he really is; others in the crowd will insist that their man is stronger and claims and counter-claims will be made.

I often hear from men who are incarcerated in prisons throughout the nation. For instance, San Quentin, the famous western prison, is believed to be the most sport-minded place in the world. A weekly sports paper is published out there. They have some splendid athletes— men who could win places in national lifting contests, a man who runs a hundred yards in nine and six-tenths seconds, baseball players who could make the big leagues, football players, tumblers, hand balancers and weight lifters—particularly weight lifters. Men out there could find a place on the stage or in the circus with the tumbling, balancing and lifting feats they perform. The San Quentinites are the most rabid strength fans in the nation.

Anywhere men gather—at school, business, at work— strength and physical ability are so often the subject of con-versation. Everyone admires the strong man. Every man would like to be a strong man. Few of them are willing to put forth the effort required to make it possible for them to join the ranks of the really strong and well developed.

Stories are told in these impromptu discussions of the strength of men they know, which would put Samson, Hercules and Ajax to shame. Men right in their neighbor-hoods are so strong and prodigiously developed that men like the late Louis Gyr, or Louis Uni, the giant of France, better known as Apollon, would be dwarfed in comparison.

Sad to relate, vaudeville has become almost a thing of the past; but at times strength stars do appear in York on the stage of one of the theatres. I go to see them, and they invariably are readers of Strength and Health magazine and come out to pay me a visit. Every York County Fair has its strong men and we have become acquainted with them. Most of them are rather an honest lot, but some are prone to disparage others while greatly enlarging their own feats. A few years ago a man was here who did perform some very fine feats of strength. He had a bar bell with him which he stated weighed 385 pounds. There was a slender young man with him, apparently undeveloped, introduced as Captain Robert Flash of the United States Marines. The young man seemed to be eighteen or nineteen years of age; no man could possibly become a captain in the United States Marines, in spite of extraordinary ability, until he was somewhere in his thirties; and the young man was so shortsighted that he would have found it impossible to enlist in the army, navy or marine corps anyway. So I knew that that was prevarication number one.

The strong man went on to explain that in a few months of eating the "health food" he offered, Captain Robert Flash had developed such uncanny strength that he could lift the 385 pounds overhead with one hand. Not fast, as most men would have to do it, the barker explained, but slow, like one would curl a twenty-five pound dumbell and then slowly press it overhead. The strong man who was doing the talking had been informed that York was the strong man center of the world; that we had a great team of weight lifters here. But he took no heed. Our young lifters know that every man has to make a living and would not have interfered or publicly debated any of his statements until the barker told the assembled crowd that the bar bell Captain Robert Flash would lift overhead later in the week was so heavy that Bob Hoffman, who had tried to lift it, could not budge it from the floor. At that eight of our lifters, who were listening, went forward and each lifted the weight overhead with one hand not once but many times. It probably weighed 170 pounds which was easy enough for champion lifters such as we have here.

But usually the men who come around to these county fairs are regular fellows. This fall the Mighty Atom was here, a man of really splendid development, fifty-eight years of age, who is in such excellent condition that he could sell anything he wanted to offer to the public. He took with him, when he left York, six hundred pounds of York weights, and is being honest with the people to whom he talks. He boosts his health food, of course, but also relates the necessity of training with weights if a man wishes to become really strong.

But what I am trying to get at with these reminiscences of a long and, at times, quite stormy career on the edge of and in the midst of strong manism, is the fact that everyone is interested in, usually to the point of admiring or loving, a strong man. A "strong man" always excites a great deal of interest and curiosity. If he is a wrestler, there will always be a crowd of young men hanging around the door to the dressing room to see him at closer quarters as he goes in and out. If he is appearing on the stage, there is always a group at the stage door, and if he is a travelling strong man, after every performance a crowd of fellows will cluster around and ask him questions. I have similar experiences every time I appear at a demonstration of lifting, strength feats or a lecture on the acquisition of strength and development. There is always a crowd around during any lull in the conversation. I am pleased to answer the many questions presented, and only sorry that I can't personally talk to more of the people who are interested.

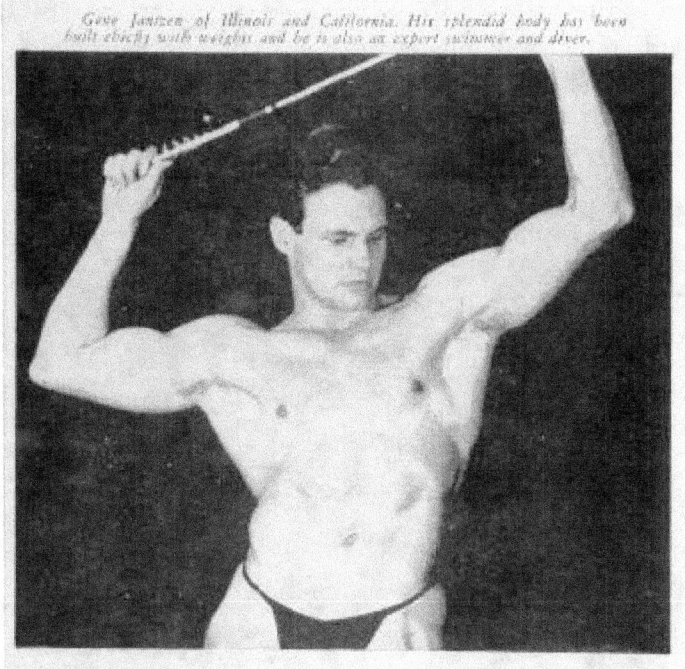

A "strong man" on the road holds a continual reception. In every town that he visits the local weight lifters and physical culturists in general will seek him out, asking for an introduction, for his autograph or for a signed photo. And always the conversation veers around to, "How did you get so strong, Mr. So and So?"—a hard question to answer, for the lifetime of work which has led up to the acquisition of the magnificent muscular development and the strength possessed by any professional strong men cannot be explained in a few minutes.

While the average uninitiated young man believes that strong men are born that way, deep down in the hearts of most of them is the belief that if he could only learn the secret, get the authentic inside information, he too could become one of the strongest men in the land. Most of the secret is first of all aspiration, then perspiration. The best methods must be adopted and followed, but hard work, by which I mean hard training, is the most important rule.

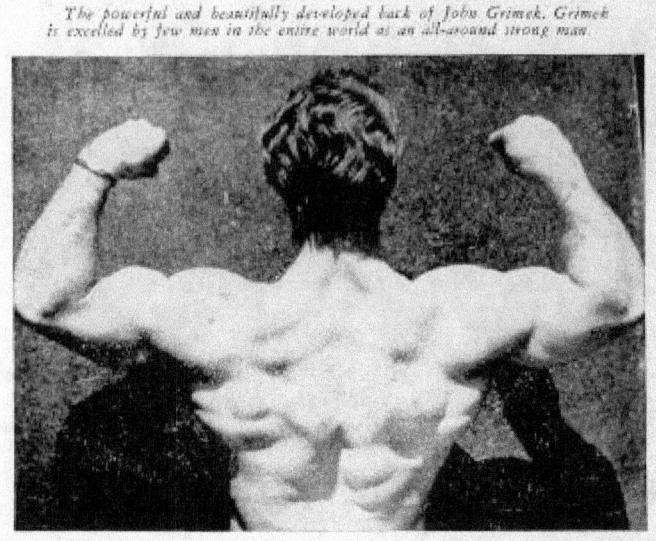

The powerful and beautifully developed back of John Grimek. Grimek is excelled by few men in the entire world as an all-around strong man.

In ten years of intensive competition and teaching of weight lifting and body building, an estimated number of 600,000 men have followed my system of training and I fully believe that at least 100,000 of these men have written to me personally asking me to outline a course for them which would make them as strong as possible in as short a time as possible. It's just as natural for a young man to wish to be powerfully developed and tremendously strong as it is for a girl to wish to be beautiful both in face and form. I'm pleased so much interest is displayed by the young men of today but it's just as impossible for me to tell them how to become strong in a single letter as it would be for Jesse Owens, who won four gold medals at the Olympics of 1936, to tell them how he trained to win those medals, or for Jack Dempsey to tell them in a letter how he became champion of the world.

My chief reason for writing this book is to try to tell these scores of thousands of interested fellows all I can about becoming strong and building an admiration-creating figure. This book gives me an opportunity to offer information, advice and instruction additional to that which has been offered in my courses and other books. It would be fine if I had the opportunity to talk personally for an hour or two to all of my pupils, but, of course, that is not possible. I meet many of them around at lifting contests, and an ever-increasing number find their way to York, where I have the opportunity to talk over their training problems. Scores of thousands have written to me, but it is certainly not possible to tell them as completely how to train and what they can expect from their training in a letter or two as it is through the writing of this book. Therefore I hope that the contents of this volume will be a means of showing the way to the strength and development-seeking youth of our country and other nations.

When a man first starts his training it is best to follow the courses exactly as they are offered. But there comes a time after the first few weeks or months when one part of the body has forged ahead of another, is better developed, so that the body builder desires to specialize in the development of the part that is lacking. The first few months of exercise may seem to be at times monotonous and tiresome, but this foundation work must be experienced to rear a structure of really great strength. Bar bell and dumbell courses and courses of cable training are so designed that every group of muscles—usually every individual muscle— will receive attention with beneficial developmental effect. The preliminary training, following the exercises of the regular courses, is designed to strengthen and to shape the muscles of the entire body, to promote a feeling of health and well being, through the improvement or stimulation of the internal organs, glands and processes.

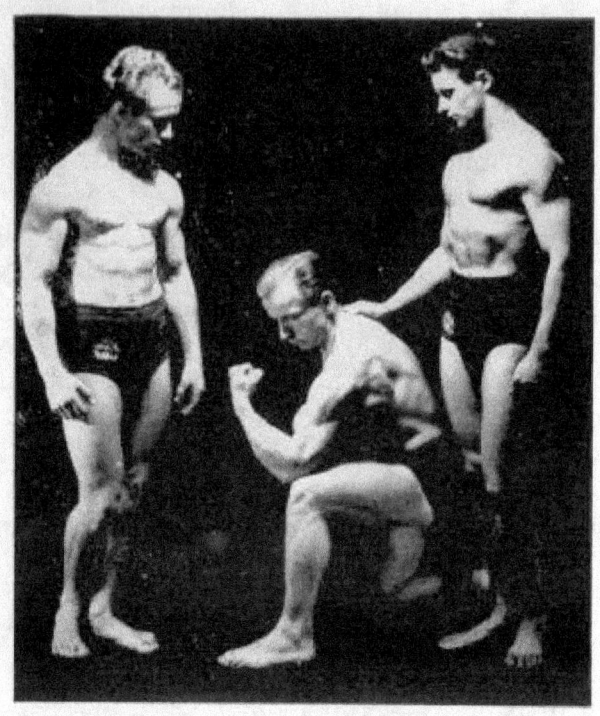

Three members of Fritsche's Gym in Philadelphia. Left to right: John Fritsche, former 112-pound senior national weight lifting champion, who weighs 140 pounds in this photo. John Stolarski who was placed second in his class in the "Best developed man contest" of York in 1939. Bob Moran, who has won championships in the 112, 118, and 126-pound classes and now is a good performer in the 148-pound division.

To really succeed in physical training, to acquire strength two or three times that of the average man, to build a beautiful figure which would do justice to a sculptor who wished to use it as a model for a statue of a Greek god, requires special training, patience, stick-to-itiveness and training knowledge—particularly training knowledge. There are many young men whose gains were infinitesimally small while they trained in a haphazard manner, without a well- prepared course of training, who made rapid, almost astounding gains when following one of my proven courses of training.

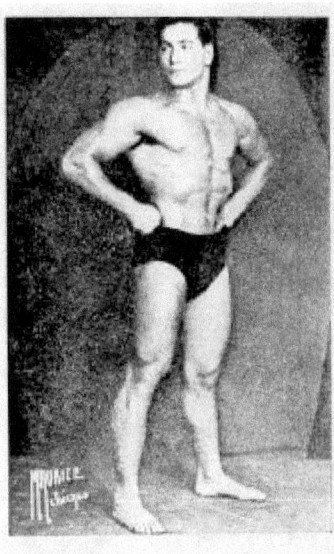

Phil Grueber, of Chicago, a former competitor in the national weight lifting championships, has since been a leading performer in professional wrestling throughout the middle west. Bar bell built muscles permit their owner to succeed at his chosen sport or physical endeavor.

Some young men fail to make haste slowly. They want to train every day; they become enthusiastic about it and find it hard to keep away from their training equipment. But it must be remembered that there is more to developing strength and a fine physique than the exercises alone. If your body is to grow steadily—to develop from the undeveloped state of the average man to the terrifically powerful physique, the beautifully-shaped body of the leading strength stars of the day—men like Grimek, Stanko, Venables, Harrison, Terpak, Terlazzo, Terry, Davis and others—you must learn to regulate your mode of living so that there is the proper balance between exercise, sleep, rest, relaxation, and proper nourishment. Follow the four major rules of health. Proper exercise, sufficient rest or sleep, good food of considerable variety at mealtimes only, and the maintenance of a tranquil mind are these few simple but all-important rules. If you are to make demands upon the muscles through heavy training, those demands must be met with proper building material, proper food, plenty of rest between training sessions so that the muscles have the opportunity to rebuild themselves after enforced exertion.

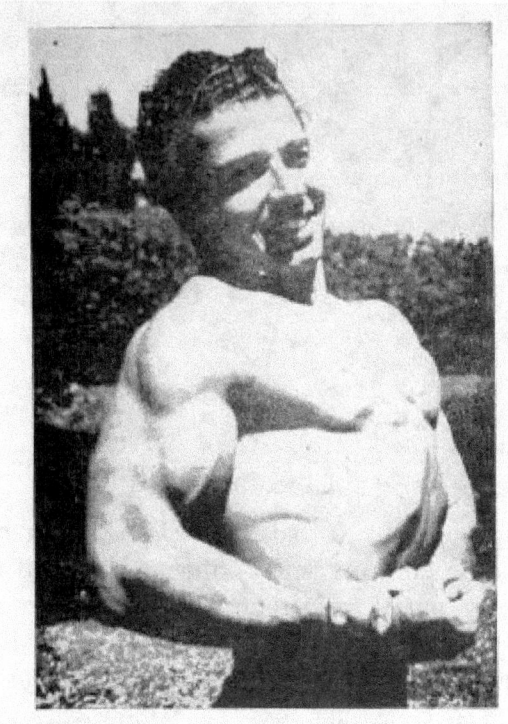

Connie Bulfin of Florida, who overcame a serious adverse physical condition to develop the splendid physique shown here.

The entire topic of acquiring superhealth, great strength and a well-muscled and proportioned body is a long subject. In this book and a number of other books I will not be able to tell you all of it in spite of the fact that I intend to try to touch on all important subjects which are factors in developing strength. For the average man, just following one of the well-designed courses will bring him all he wants; but for the man who seeks the limit in building strength and muscle, a much deeper study of the subject is necessary.

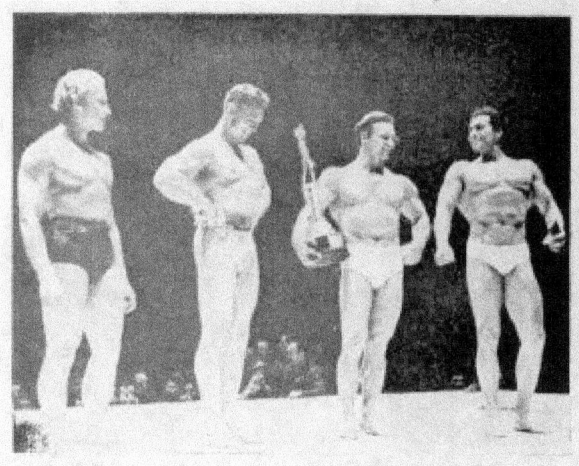

The finalists in the most representative Mr. America contest of them all. Held in Madison Square Garden, in conjunction with the national weight lifting championships, it brought out America's best built men in great numbers. Left to right is Ludwig Schusterich, winner of the title Mr. New York, before his seventeenth birthday. He is an ambitious weight lifter and member of the famous Cooper A. C. of Brooklyn. Finished 3rd in the great contest. Frank (Leight) Stepanek, powerful New York policeman who was placed second. John Grimek, the winner of the Mr. America title as well as the Most Muscular Man in America and best developed arm titles, and Chick Deutch of Brooklyn, N. Y., who was placed 4th.

Few if any men have had the opportunity I have had to learn the training methods of the champions in strength and development. I was always interested in strength, athletics and well-developed men. I believe my interest started as early as four years. I religiously followed my first "train you by mail" course when I was ten years of age, and through all my life I have intensely followed athletics and physical training. I have been inquisitive and have spent years in asking questions. Often I was one of the young men waiting at the stage door to see the great strength athlete. For many years before I started my own professional career I hunted up strong men, both professional and amateur, at their homes when I happened to be working in the city in which they lived. I followed weight lifting and weight lifters through nearly every state of the Union. Since the beginning of organized weight lifting in this country I have not missed an important championship.

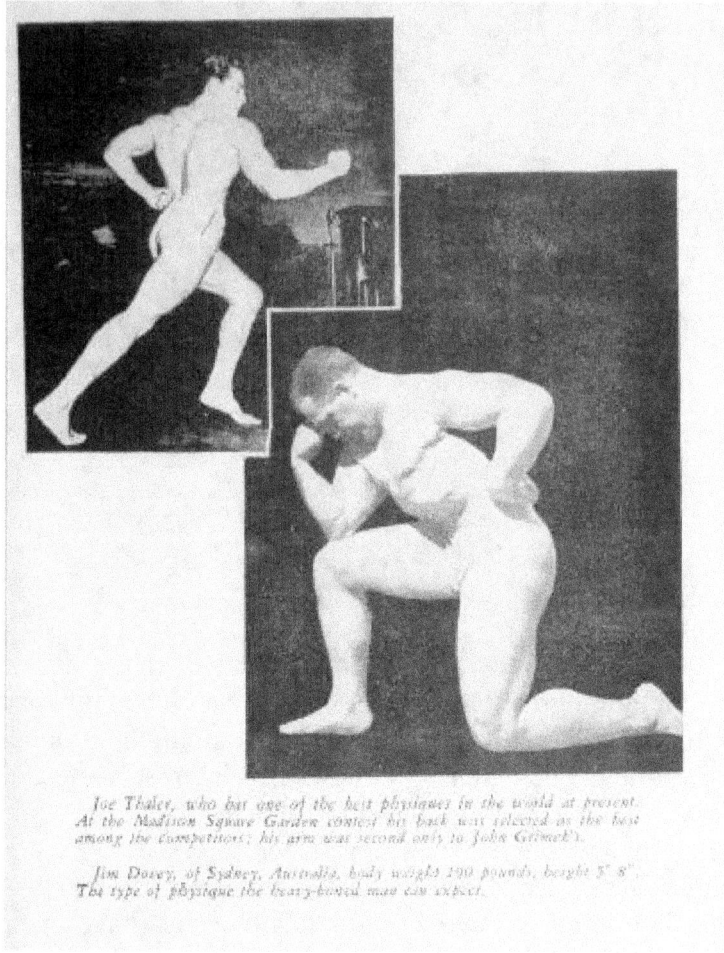

Joe Thaler, who has one of the best physiques in the world at present. At the Madison Square Garden contest his back was selected as the best among the competitors; his arm was second only to John Grimek's.

Jim Dorey, of Sydney, Australia, body weight 190 pounds, height 5' 8". The type of physique the heavy-boned man can extest.

The Olympic Games always find me present trying to see all the events from the gymnastics at 6 a. m. through the afternoon rowing, the evening boxing, wrestling, and weight lifting until 4 a. m. or later. I try to see everything, talk to everyone, and read a great deal besides. I have been

16

doing this for a moderate lifetime, so have come to know personally most of the amateur and professional strength athletes (by strength athletes I mean weight lifters, wrestlers, balancers, tumblers, and strong men in general) of the last score of years. I doubt if any other man knows more of them than I do.

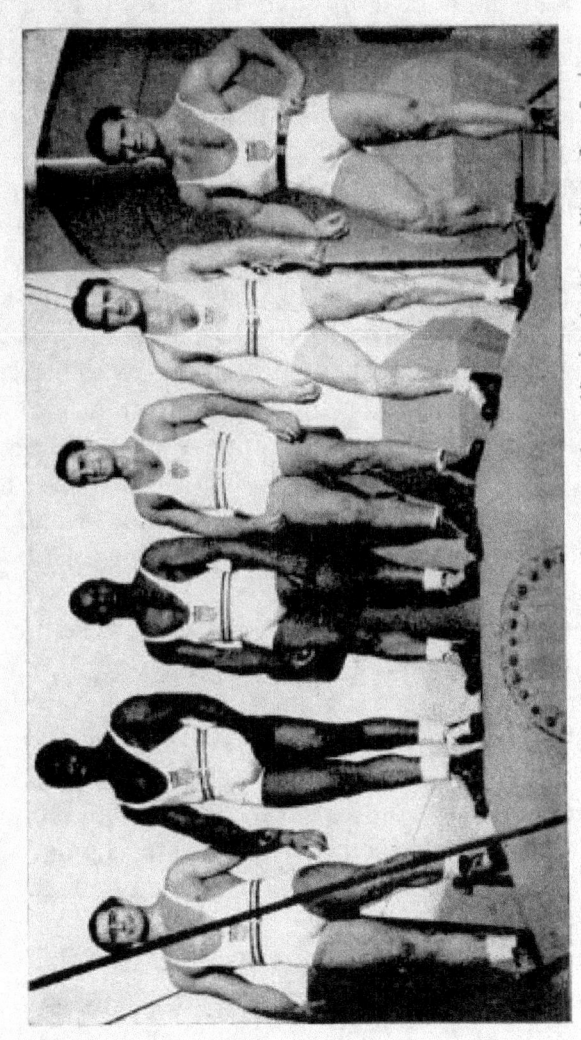

The United States champions of 1939 and 1940 on their way to the world's championships in Vienna: Steve Stanko, heavyweight; John Davis, just 17 years of age who won to win the world's championship; John Terry, 132-pound champion who set an official world's two hands snatch record; Tony Terlazzo, Olympic champion of 1936, world's champion of '37 and '38; Terpak, 165-pound world's champion, and John Grimek, who was champion of North America.

I constantly train myself and daily associate with a group of young champions who hold all the United States and most of the world's records in the standard lifts and totals of those lifts. I live right in the midst of the strength and health center of the world. I literally breathe, eat, think and sometimes sleep weight lifting, strength and development. I have learned a great deal through the men I have met; I have seen my theories proven on my own body and that of my many pupils or the members of my own team of strong men. All in all I believe I am qualified to write with authority concerning every angle of the strongman world. My team, which I have personally coached, has become the world's best. I have continued to improve myself each year (best proven by a one hand lift overhead bent press style of 202 on my thirty-eighth birthday, 220 on my thirty-ninth birthday, 263½ on my fortieth birthday, 270 on my forty-first birthday). I am sure that if you will follow the advice I offer, without dividing your time and effort trying what others tell you, you will obtain as fine results as the great group of York strong men have acquired. In the past there have been instructors who did not practice what they reached, men who had never proven with their own bodies that their training methods were correct. And today we have a similar condition. Most of the people who are selling bar bells and dumbells are ashamed to show a picture of their own physiques. They have ruined their own physiques through faulty training methods or have not succeeded in building a body that they dare to show as a physique photo. What results do you expect to obtain from men who have not proven the correctness of their teachings? Over ten thousand testimonial letters, unsolicited letters, have been received and placed on my desk for my personal attention here in York. The most amazing cases of physical rejuvenation, of the acquisition of great strength and development from a very mediocre beginning, are received each week. It's a pleasure to be in this work, helping others reach the limit in strength, health, and development.

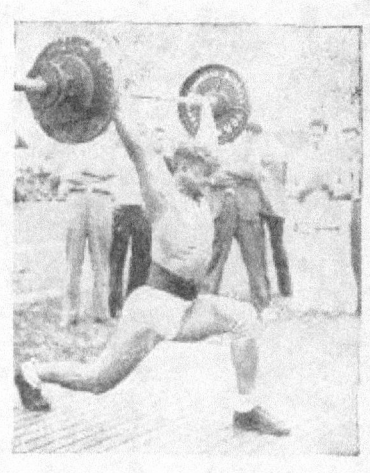

Bob Brinker, of the Twin City Weight Lifting Club, Easton, Pa., one of the nation's leading light heavyweight lifters. Like all star weight lifters, he is magnificently developed as well as strong. His best lifting records are: press 235, snatch 265, jerk 310.

There is sufficient in my regular courses for the average individual who is satisfied to be two or three times as strong as the average undeveloped man—to be just well built— but this book will contain advanced information and instruction to help the man who has already made progress reach the championship class. This type of man has already tasted the joys of superhealth and great strength. He's learned the admiration his strength and muscle have engendered in the minds of his friends and acquaintances; he's found it a means of attaining greater satisfaction and joy from life; he's heard the favorable comments from friends and strangers alike who see him at the pool or the bathing beach. He longs to go farther, to take rank with the best built and strongest men in the land. He desires to be a weight lifter, a strong man, to be an artist's model perhaps, operate his own gymnasium, be a physical education teacher, a professional wrestler, boxer, or acrobat, he earnestly craves to reach the heights. This book will serve best for that type of superenthusiastic young man.

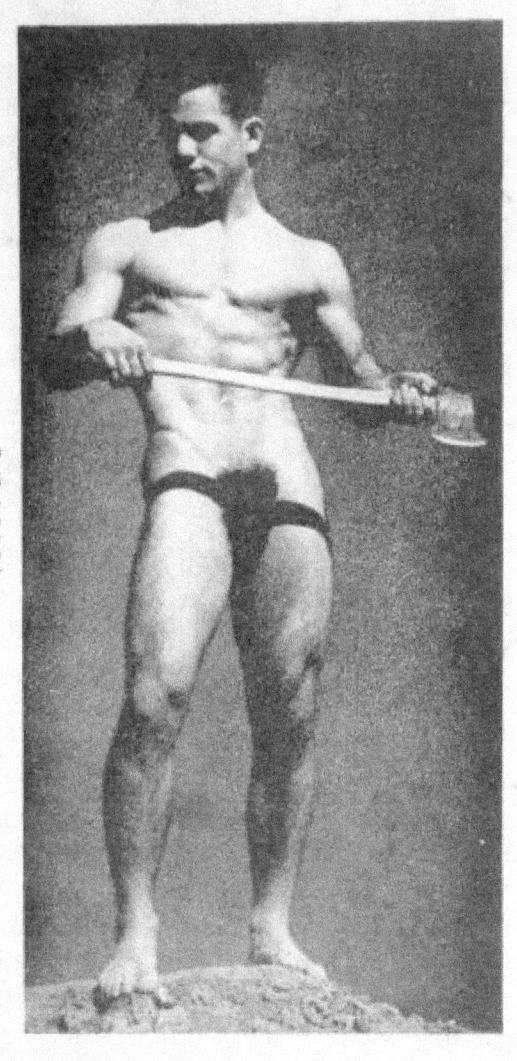

A splendid pose by a little-known weight lifter, Vernon H. Schwenke, of Milwaukee, Wis. The pose is original and illustrates the results which can be obtained in a few months of training with the proper methods.

I wish to disclose the best way the average young man can follow to become stronger; to prove to him that he can become a great deal stronger and better built than he would expect. I wish to prove that if he follows the advice the pages to come will present, he will develop permanent strength, build powerful internal works which will make him not only live more fully but live longer.

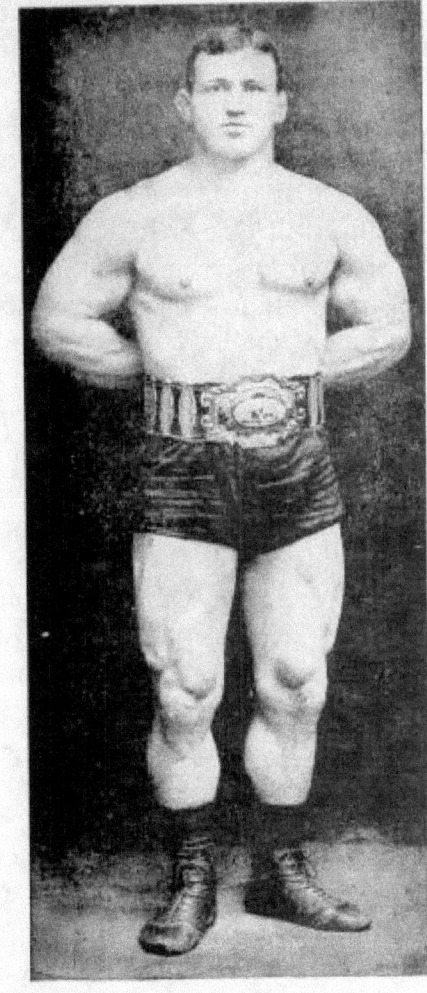

John Lemm of Switzerland, the possessor of one of the most powerfully developed physiques in the annals of weight training. Former holder of European championships and records, he is now one of the famous Swiss Alpine guides.

I hope to prove that strength is possible for any fellow, that even those who are apparently helplessly crippled have built a great measure of strength through proper training methods. Those who are lacking in size, in strength, vigor, or who suffer from minor diseases can first of all overcome these conditions through the medium of corrective developing and invigorating exercises, and then after this preliminary work has been done can acquire that stage of great strength and superdevelopment which is the crowning glory of true manhood.

I have seen so many weaklings become strong men and champion strength athletes that I am convinced the ability to become strong is within all of us. In the many years during which I have been editor-in-chief of Strength and Health magazine, we have published an ever-increasing number of articles about men who have overcome all forms of physical injuries or irregularities. In fact most of our strength stars of today, the men who hold the records and have won the championships, made their beginning in physical training because they were extremely weak or actually ailing in some manner. Too seldom is the man who is naturally strong willing to train to become a champion; he is prone to be satisfied. The men who suffer from some form of physical inferiority are the men who become the champions; they first overcome the condition which torments them and then go on to be the strongest and the best-built men in the land.

The records have proven that any man, regardless of his present condition, whether fat, thin, weak, ailing or crippled, can, with persistence, ambition and knowledge, improve himself and revolutionize his entire life.

Strong men of today are of all shapes, sizes, types and designs, of all nationalities and of several colors. No nation, race, or color has a monopoly on strength, as you will perceive as you continue with this book. Every race and color has its strong men. It is the life that is led, the training methods which are employed which contribute to a man's strength. There are strong men who are well over six feet —others scarcely more than five feet, some are large-boned, others small-boned. With these two extremes and all the classes in between are to be found men who possess that distinctive beauty of form and high degree of muscular development which marks the true "strong man." Physical power and development are within the reach of any man who will strive faithfully to attain his physical desires.

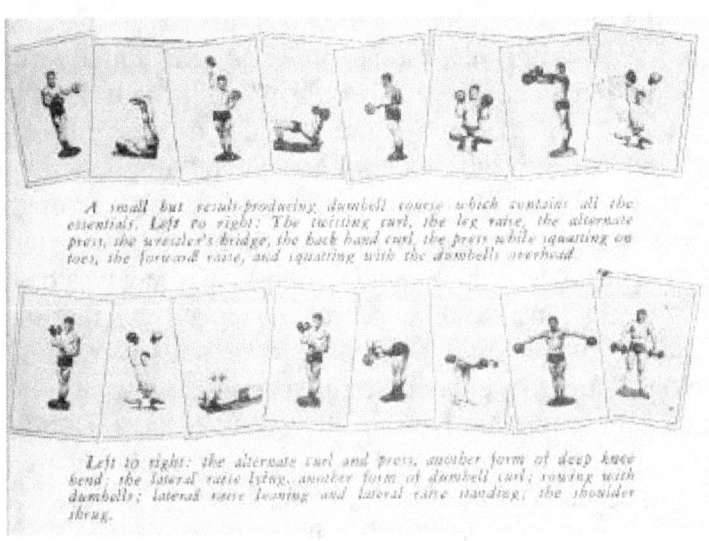

A small but result-producing dumbell course which contains all the essentials. Left to right: The twisting curl, the leg raise, the alternate press, the wrestler's bridge, the back hand curl, the press while squatting on toes, the forward raise, and squatting with the dumbells overhead.

Left to right: the alternate curl and press, another form of deep knee bend; the lateral raise lying, another form of dumbell curl; rowing with dumbells; lateral raise leaning and lateral raise standing; the shoulder shrug.

CHAPTER TWO
Can Strength Be Acquired?

How did the strong men become strong? is a question frequently asked. Were they born that way, or was it the result of training? There is such a thing as inherited strength. We have it in the animal kingdom in the powerful, heavily muscled bulldog. If a bulldog spends its life confined within the limits of a short chain, it is still a mighty animal. Most of its power is the result of heredity. A greyhound will be tall, long and slender even though it should be trained as a sled dog. It will become some stronger and more heavily muscled but still it will not approach the bulldog in strength. The heavy draft horse is big and powerful even though it has never been hitched to the wagon or the plow. It has inherited strength, while a racing horse, whose ancestors for many generations have been bred for speed, by intelligent mating of its parents, by proper care and exercise, has developed superbly shapely, steel-spring-like muscles, but it is slender in comparison to the draft horse. Bulldogs, greyhounds, draft horses and rac- ing thoroughbreds are not products of nature but of careful, painstaking and intelligent selection over a period of hundreds of years. Skilled breeders have developed all the types of domestic animals we have today—the Holstein, Guernsey or Ayrshire cattle; the Percheron, Clydesdale, or thoroughbred horses; the Great Dane, the Scotch terrier, the Russian Wolfhound; the Jersey white giant, the largest among the chickens, which attains a weight of thirteen or fourteen pounds, and the cocky but tiny bantam which weighs scarcely more than a pound.

In most quarters animals are bred with the greatest of care as to handling and feeding, while the same stock raisers permit their own children to grow up in the most haphazard manner. There would be a far better race of people if a fraction of the attention, knowledge and care, which result in the thoroughbred or pedigreed farm animal, were directed toward the development of better humans.

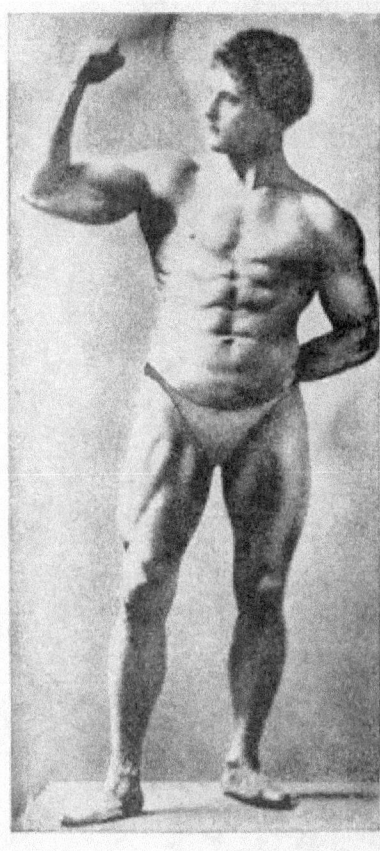

Eugene Sandow when 19 years of age. About the time he was wrestling in Italy. Although his physique improved greatly with each passing year, he had already attained near physical perfection at this time.

Many experiments have been conducted with animals which of course are not possible with humans. Five hundred generations of rats extend only over a period of twenty-five years owing to their rapid maturity. Five hundred generations of humans would require approximately ten thousand years, but in just a few generations of breeding humans by careful selection, as is done with animals, we could have any sort of an individual desired—an early-maturing, long- living class of men who would weigh five hundred pounds in the best of condition; or a race of small men weighing less than fifty pounds who would reach an age of senility at the present normal period of maturity. Careful selection for the particular type or characteristics desired would bring these results as has been done by man in the breeding of animals.

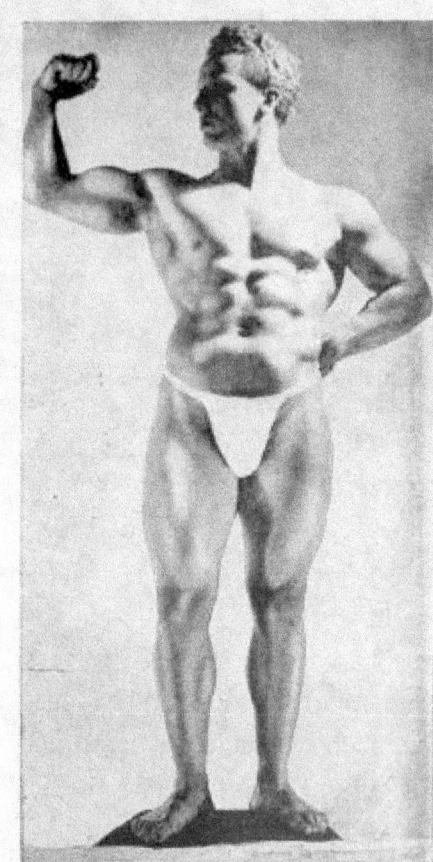

Phil Campau of New York City. This recent photo of the little known New York City youth, 19 years of age at the time of taking photo, compares even more than favorably with that of Sandow above on the opposite page. Campau is an all around barbell man and was one of the contestants in the Annual Best Press championships of America. His record in this style of lifting is 225.

Returning from an exhibition of weight lifting in Cleveland last year, we had fun for over two hundred miles discussing the breeding of champion weight lifters. It was explained at great length just how we would obtain rapid maturity, so that in the several generations the weight lifting breeder could expect to live the type desired would be obtained. We talked of breeding two kinds of weight lifters —the type with long backs and short legs, who are stars at the squat style of lifting, usually short in the arms and good pressers; and another type with long legs and short backs who would possess favorable leverage in pulling weights to the shoulder and overhead, and the proper ratio of shoulder width in proportion to length of the upper and lower arm which would create a good presser. We were to "line breed" for two or three generations and then "cross breed" these two distinct types and thus obtain the perfect weight lifter— a heavyweight, weighing not less than 300 pounds in good condition, a man who would combine all the desirable features which would put the records up past the point of imagination at the present time.

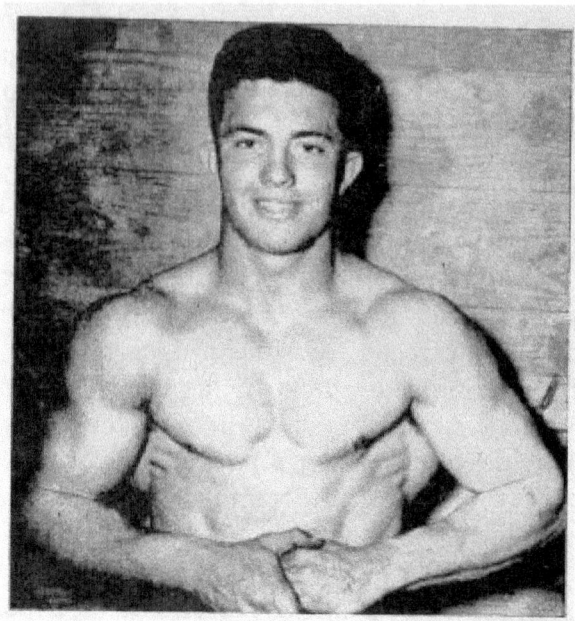

Fred Ross of Moberly, Mo. A star football player who built the
physique shown in this photo, chiefly with weights. He has found that
weight training gives him more speed, power, drive, and all-around football playing ability.

Another unknown who has suddenly blossomed forth with one of the
best physiques which could ever grace a human body. Thousands of
weight-trained men who never even have a photo taken have built physiques
which rival the very best. This photo is of Joe Lauriano of Honolulu.

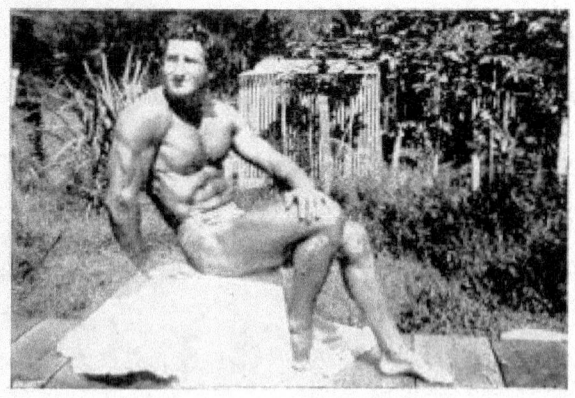

But this will never be done. Eugenics will not marry eugenics. The young man will marry the first trim-waisted, sparkling-eyed, vivacious and lovely little lady he falls in love with. He'll probably meet this girl by accident—perhaps on a picnic, at his place of business, at a dance, or in some foreign country as was the case with the soldiers who went to France, Germany, Italy or Russia during the Great War. He won't be interested in how long her parents lived, what they died of, whether in her germ plasm there is the possibility of cancer, heart trouble, tuberculosis, kidney disease or many other of the diseases which are considered to a large extent to be inherited. The boy will marry the girl he likes without the slightest thought of the offspring which will result from that union. In the majority of cases unlikes attract; the little lady likes the big man, the big man likes the little woman. The small man likes a big woman and vice versa. We have the case of John L. Sullivan, America's first great boxing champion, whose father was quite average in size and whose mother was huge and strong. We learn that Louis Cyr, considered by many to be "the strongest man who ever lived," had a huge Amazonlike mother and an average-sized father. Louis weighed nearly four hundred pounds later in life, yet he selected a lady to be Madame Cyr who weighed less than a hundred pounds. One of Cyr's favorite feats of strength later in life was apparently performed in an impromptu manner. He would be leaning across the bar of the tavern he kept after he retired from active competition in the world of weights, and from the living quarters in the back of the tavern would appear Madame Cyr dressed in her best "go-to-town clothes"; without removing one elbow from the bar, Cyr would reach back with the other hand. Mrs. Cyr would seat herself upon the huge palm, and with an elevator or escalator-like service, Louis would lift her across the counter and set her down gently on the other side. It was not to be expected that the offspring of a mating from such divergent types would be very large or very strong. There are many others who will swear, argue and even fight over their belief that Louis Uni, the giant of old France, better known as Apollon, was the strongest man who ever lived. He Was a giant in size, and approached a body weight of 300 pounds in later life. But he too was enamored by and married one of these vitriolic little ladies who completely dominated him in rather shameful fashion throughout their lives together. Madame Uni weighed less than a hundred pounds.

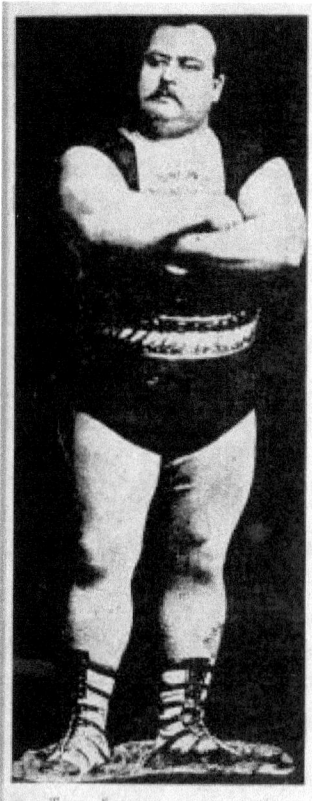

Tony Sansone, a contrasting type to Cyr, with a physique which is much admired. In this photo he is 6 feet tall and weighs approximately 180 pounds.

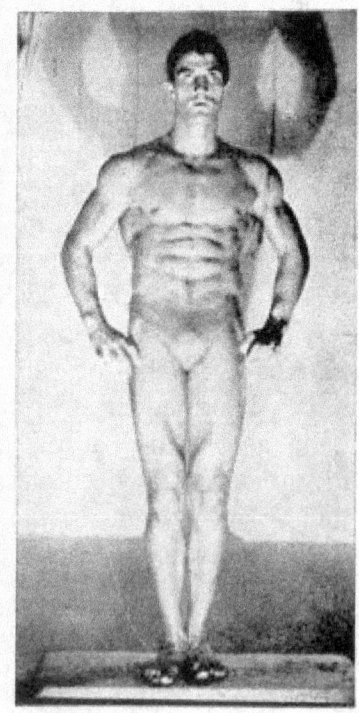

Louis Cyr, freely considered to be the strongest man who ever lived. As he appeared in this photo he weighs 315 pounds, and had just exceeded Eugene Sandow's world's one hand press record of 269, with his own hoist of 273.

It's nature's way to balance the human race and to prevent the development of a race of giants or dwarfs. Seldom in the history of mankind has there been a definite attempt to produce gigantic men. It has been done for hundreds of years with Oriental wrestlers, particularly in Japan and India. In these countries where small, slight men are the average citizen there are four-hundred-pound wrestlers who grunt, push and pull with all the power and abandon of a huge water buffalo. For centuries the wrestlers have been a separate group or clan; only the biggest of the wrestlers' sons can follow in the fathers' footsteps and become wrestlers. Only these wrestlers are permitted to marry the daughters of other famous wrestlers. That's selective breeding applied to humans and the result we see in the huge and powerful Oriental wrestlers so dear to the hearts of their countrymen.

But most of us are of such mixed ancestry; our ancestors only two generations back possess such a conglomeration of characteristics that few of us know what to expect. In my own case, for instance, my maternal grandparents are Irish and Scotch, and my paternal grandparents Swiss and English. I know considerable about the family trees of these ancestors, but this tells me nothing. I know that my paternal grandfather, who died at ninety-seven, the oldest child in his family, has seven brothers and sisters still living. Yet his son, my father, died at fifty-six. I know that my maternal grandfather's brothers and relatives were quite tall, some of them being six feet seven; yet one uncle, the first offspring of this union, is not over five feet six inches tall, while I in the next generation am six feet three, and the tallest in my immediate family. Some of my people apparently died of old age, an occasional one from tuberculosis, cancer, or heart trouble. How am I to know what I might die of? I may be hanged for all I know, may live to a hundred as some of my ancestors did or die when little past middle age as some other relatives have done. Of course there is this difference: I want to live long. I appreciate this world and I follow the rules of living which will promote longer than normal life.

If you who read this will consider your own ancestors, it will be evident that you cannot know what to expect. It would be simple indeed if humans knew what to anticipate as we know what to expect from a study of the Mendelian laws of heredity. When we breed a white rabbit and a black rabbit, it has been proven that over a sufficient number of generations the resulting offspring from this union of the black rabbit and the white rabbit will produce the following percentage of offspring: one white rabbit, one black rabbit and two brown rabbits. If these white rabbits are bred with each other, only white rabbits will result, and if the black rabbits are mated, only black rabbits will be produced. But if the two brown rabbits are mated once again we go back to our former ratio of one white rabbit, one black rabbit and two brown rabbits.

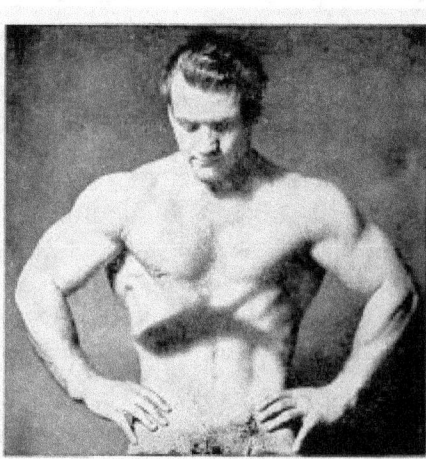

John Grimek again. John Grimek rightfully deserves the title he won at Madison Square Garden, "Most Muscular Man in America." He has huge shapely limbs, a large rounded, deep chest, broad powerful shoulders and a waist so slender it is almost wasp like in comparison. In this photo his waist is less in circumference than his thigh.

Or if two types of sweet peas are grafted together, the resulting peas will never be intermediate in size but will be tall or short in a direct proportion, which has been proven time and again to be the result of the Mendelian theory.

To a great extent humans can disregard their heredity in considering their possibilities in developing strength and muscle. I say to a great extent, for it is to be expected that strong fathers and mothers will produce strong sons. But so many physical attributes are contained in our ancestry that we hardly know what to expect. Seldom is the son of a great runner as fast as his father, although speed is an inherited characteristic; seldom is the son of a great strong man as powerful as his father, usually because he has mated with a—to him—attractive woman who does not have powerful ancestors; and just as rarely is the son of any other great athlete as good as his father. And, similarly, great strong men and outstanding athletes spring up in families where the parents have apparently not been athletic. Let us consider some of the great young weight lifters and strong men of the present: Steve Stanko, the present heavyweight United States lifting champion, who just a day prior to the writing of this chapter broke the world's record in the two hands clean and jerk lift by hoisting 371 pounds to arm's length overhead, officially. His case would seem to be one of heredity. He came from sturdy stock, his father being known as one of the strongest men in the district from which Steve originally hailed. His grandfather died recently in Budapest and had been famed throughout his life for his great strength. Yet Steve grew up to six feet in height, 145 pounds in body weight, athletic enough to be selected as All State Fullback, but hardly stronger than the average. It was only when he took up the practice of weight lifting that he rapidly became the superman he is today. His heredity must have served him in good stead for he gained more rapidly than any man I know. After two years of irregular training he entered official competition, winning, in his first year's competition, in turn the state championship, the district championship, the junior national championship, the senior national championship, the championship of North America, and placed second in the world's championship in Vienna.

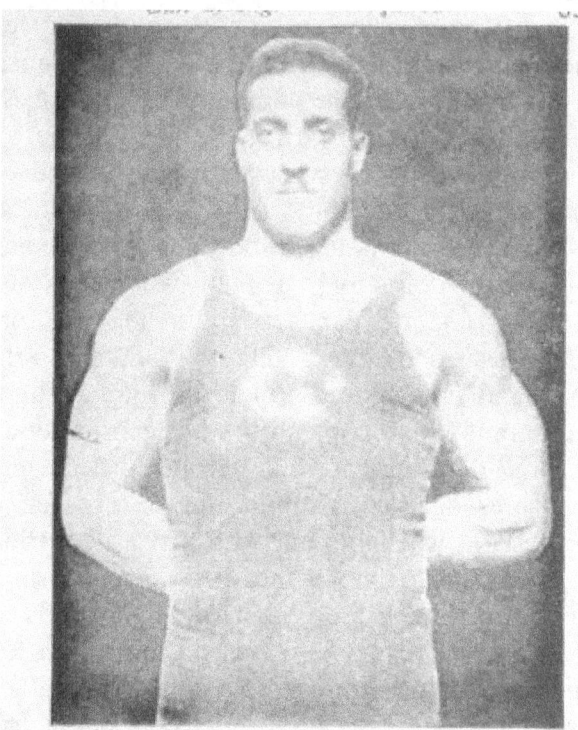

El Said Nosseir, the first of the great Egyptian weight lifters. He started the world by winning the 182-pound title at the Olympics of 1928. In this photo he is a 181 class man, later he became the world's best weight lifter, pressing 235 pounds, two hands snatching 275 and cleaning and jerking 368.

In this latter competition he made the highest two hands snatch and the highest clean and jerk of any of the world's mighty lifters who were in that competition. He has continued to improve and has gained fifty pounds in this last year in his two hands press alone. I believe that heredity played an important part in Steve's rapid rise to the

34

heights of the strength world, but if he had not trained he would have been no different from many thousands of other young men in this country. His bbdy was like the fertile field I sometimes write about, the field of fertile soil which, when plowed, harrowed and planted, then cultivated, produces a bumper crop. In contrast there are others who have not inherited the sound, perfectly operating internal organs who will not progress so rapidly. They are like the field of more or less impoverished soil which must be plowed, fertilized and although cultivated more than the first field will not produce a similar crop until years of attention make of it a fertile field. A longer period of training is required for some men until they have made the important internal changes which make it possible for them to gain in weight, height, strength and muscular development.

And John Grimek. There's a man who most people believe must be a product of heredity. But I've met his people a number of times, and although it must be admitted that they come of sturdy, central European stock, they are no different from thousands of other families. John's older brother bought the first bar bell in the Grimek family when John was a youngster not yet in his teens. He was interested in physical training and encouraged his little brother to wrestle with the little sister, and to try to lift weights. John trained hard at a youthful age, became much larger and stronger than any other member of his immediate family. John's elder brother looks not a bit different from millions of working men in this country. Grimek became the most muscular man of the day, perhaps of all time. With this wealth of muscles he combines a symmetry that is un-excelled. He has wisely moulded his own body. It is ad-mitted that every man even with similar training methods could not be a Grimek, for there has been no other man just like him in development and proportions. But were it not for his intelligent, persistent and proper training he would be just average in strength and development. One glance at the broad shoulders, the huge rounded chest, the phenomenally slender waist, the highly developed legs, will prove that physical training pays. Photos of Grimek don't do him justice; the man must be seen to be appreciated, although the poses of him which appear in this book give more than a faint idea of the great physique he has won for himself through proper physical training. He has everything in a physical way; was the heavyweight champion of 1936, the man who made the greatest American total at the Olympic games of 1936. He has continental pressed 326 pounds and jerked 370 pounds from the shoulder.

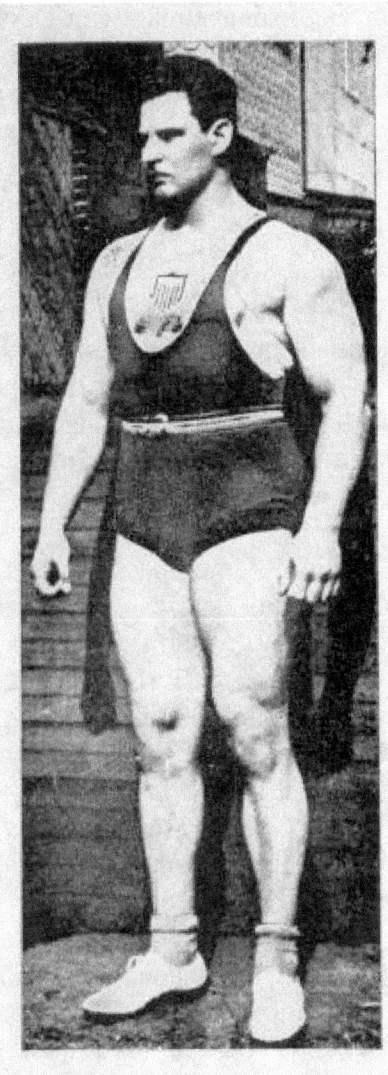

Dave Mayor at the height of his lifting career in 1937 when he was America's strongest weight lifter and national champion. He weighs 265 as he appears here and aside from other great measurements his arms stretched the tape to 19½ inches; they were the largest muscular arms in the world at that time.

I have briefly discussed the heavyweight champions of 1936, 1938, 1939 and 1940—Grimek in the former case, and Stanko these latter years. In the year of 1937 Dave Mayor was the champion. Dave came into this world as a four and one-half pound baby. I know his mother and father well. Nice people. The mother a bit taller than the average, the father a bit larger than the ordinary man. But Dave first reached his height of six feet one and a half inches, weighing 120 pounds. It was a long road from that point to the 265 pounds he weighed when he won the national heavyweight championship. At that time he had the largest muscular arms in the world, nineteen inches in circumference. He's now a professional wrestler. He has a younger brother who is going to college, about the same height, body weight 165 after a limited period of weight training. Had Dave not trained hard and persistently, three times a day, five times a week at one stage of his training, he would not have exceeded his brother in strength and development. Doesn't this seem to be another case of acquired rather than inherited strength and development?

Let's go back to the little fellows. A member of our team, in fact the oldest member of our team, is Art Levan, who won ten consecutive senior national weight lifting championships in the 126-pound class. Finally his weight grew to the point where he could no longer enter the 126-pound division. He won the 132-pound North American championship, and then he entered the 148-pound class which has been dominated by the world's champion, Tony Terlazzo. I have known Art Levan for sixteen years—when he was first starting weight lifting. He was a little fellow then, seventeen years of age, who had been encouraged to take up weight training because of a heart and nerve ailment. Even his winning of eleven national titles in a row does not fully illustrate the tremendous power this small man developed.

Next is another great champion, Dick Bachtell. Nine times he won first place in the United States championships. On three other occasions he was a place winner. He was a fat boy when he started. From this beginning he developed world's record-breaking ability in lifting, became proficient and famous as a balancer and a tumbler and is still one of the best lifters in the country. Without training he would have been a roly-poly fat man, such as are many grocery clerks.

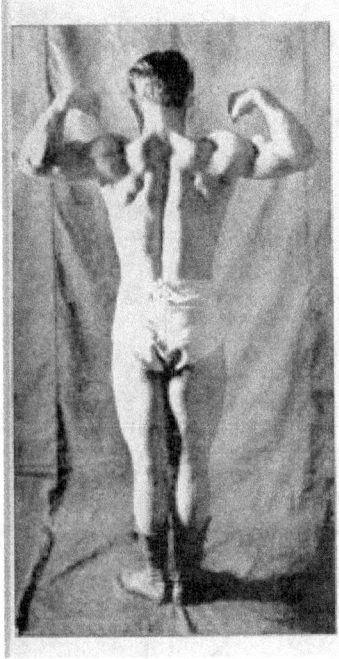
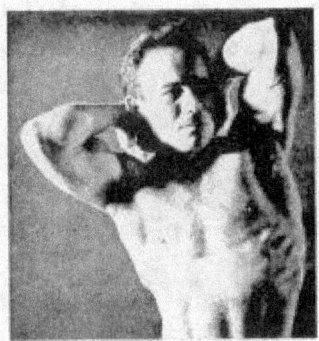

Above, Dick Bachtell, the oldest man in point of years of action, still in national competition. He won his first national title in 1928 and is much better today than in his earlier championship winning years.

Ari Levan, at a bodyweight of 126 pounds, during the period in which he was creating the unbroken string of 11 national titles, ten in the 126-pound class and one in the 132.

And now we come to what many consider the greatest of them all, Tony Terlazzo, the man who year after year wins the national and world's 148-pound championship. In 1932 he first garnered the national 132-pound United States lifting title. He slowly gained in weight and strength. In 1932 he established a United States record in the two hands press of 180½ pounds. In 1936 he established a world's record in that same class with a press of 215. Since then he has lifted in the 148-pound class and pushed the world's press record up to 255 pounds. He has made a good practice press with 265 pounds, he has elevated, in the lift known as the clean and jerk, 340 pounds to arm's length overhead, 45 pounds more than double his own body weight. At present he is the 132-pound Olympic champion, the 148-pound United States and world's champion, the 165-pound champion of North America. In the beginning he could not put seventy pounds overhead in any style with two hands. This in spite of the fact that he had long been interested in physical training and had practiced gymnastics and wrestling. He had absolutely no encouragement from his parents, in fact he succeeded in spite of their opposition. They were small and average physically. Could anyone truthfully say that the success of this great lifter is the result of anything but his own persistent and intelligent efforts?

Johnny Terpak is the United States and world's middle-weight champion. In three short years he went from an unknown as a lifter to the world's title, which he won in Paris, France. What part did heredity play in his weight lifting triumphs? Johnny grew to young manhood weighing 135 pounds. He was fond of athletics and was a halfback, sprinter and amateur fighter while in school, not unlike many thousands of high school athletes throughout our nation. When he became a member of our team here in York, he rapidly rose to the world's championship. The world's a mighty big place, and when a man is world's champion he has reached the physical heights indeed. How about John Davis? He's the lad who won the world's light heavyweight title in Vienna before he reached his eighteenth birthday. His mother is of good size and quite healthy; no doubt like most colored fellows only a few generations removed from savage ancestries where only the strongest and the fittest survived, he had a good inheritance. In his earlier contests he amassed a lifting total of 600 pounds. From that point it surged up to by far a world's record of 893 pounds in the 181-pound class; 819 and 830 have won world's titles in the past. Davis shattered the world's press record by 22½ pounds. He startled the world when he defeated the great French champion Hostin, the Olympic winner in 1932 and 1936, and when he also defeated the world's champion of 1937—Haller of Austria. Weight training made it possible for Davis to reach the heights.

There are many other men who are members of the famous York Bar Bell Lifting Club, the world's strongest weight lifting team, who are further proof that strength is acquired rather than inherited. There are many thousands of York pupils who have transformed their bodies into symmetrical powerful human machines two or three times as strong, as enduring, as the average human body. There is even my own case to add more proof to the fact that training is far more important than heredity in the acquisition of strength. I weighed 140 pounds when I first reached my present height of six feet three inches. After years of participation in most forms of athletics and games, I weighed 180 pounds when I first learned of bar bell training. I had won approximately five hundred prizes in various forms of athletics—had won championships both district and national in a wide variety of sports. I was victor in these events through determination, skill, endurance, the ability to drive myself to the point of collapse rather than through strength, for I was not strong when I first started weight training. I could not press 80 pounds overhead. It was only after months of training that I became strong enough and sufficiently skilled to lift sixty-five pounds overhead with one hand. When I see the average untrained man so easily press fifty pounds overhead with one hand, or see some girl or woman lift a hundred pounds overhead with two hands, then do I fully realize how lacking in strength I was in the beginning.

One day little Gracie Bard, one of the Strength and Health models, was posing on our lawn for some bar bell exercises.

41

She had curled in turn forty, fifty and sixty pounds. Our colored maid was watching and I said, "Del, do you think you could do that?" She said, "I don't know, but I'll try." Sixty pounds was ridiculously easy for her. I had to remember that I could not curl sixty pounds when I started. I loaded the bar to eighty pounds and she curled it just as easily and pressed it overhead without changing the grip of her hands which meant that she was pressing the most difficult way. It was done with absurd ease—a demonstration which proved rather forcefully to me that anything I possess in the way of strength is the result of training.

It has long been my theory, and I am endeavoring to prove it by being a human guinea pig, that a man can continue to improve from his earliest youth until he reaches the age of at least fifty. Then he can remain near the top for long additional years. I saw Schillburg, the Austrian weight lifter, a man of fifty-two years of age, who was still good enough to become a member of his country's Olympic weight lifting team, press 286 pounds. He's not such a big man either. I had to remember that John Y. Smith, of Boston, weight 160 pounds, a few years ago had proven himself to be the strongest man in all New England; that Oscar Mathes at seventy-seven can still perform the feats of his youth; that Warren Lincoln Travis, performing at Coney Island, past sixty years of age, is defying the world to equal his feats of strength. Otto Arco was here last week; he became the most muscular man of his time, the possessor of a seventeen and a quarter inch arm on his 140 pound body, and he still has an arm of that size. He continued to improve from his early youth until past fifty. He showed a picture of himself taken when he was sixteen years of age and although he had already made a good start, he was certainly not a phenomenon. I have continued to improve through the years although I travel considerably and have little training time, and in spite of a multitude of duties. I do not claim to be a strong man, but I have acquired more than my share of strength and health. Each year I have made encouraging gains which is the best proof that strength is acquired rather than inherited. An improvement in strength and technique made it possible for me to gain from the 65 pound one arm lift of my first year in training to a recent 270 pounds.

All the great amount of illustrations and proof I could offer point to one true fact—that training is more important than heredity in acquiring strength. I believe that it is within the possibilities and the capabilities of every man to make a very marked improvement in his physical attributes providing he will devote at least a fraction of the time at improving his body that is required to become proficient at mechanical work, professional or business vocations.

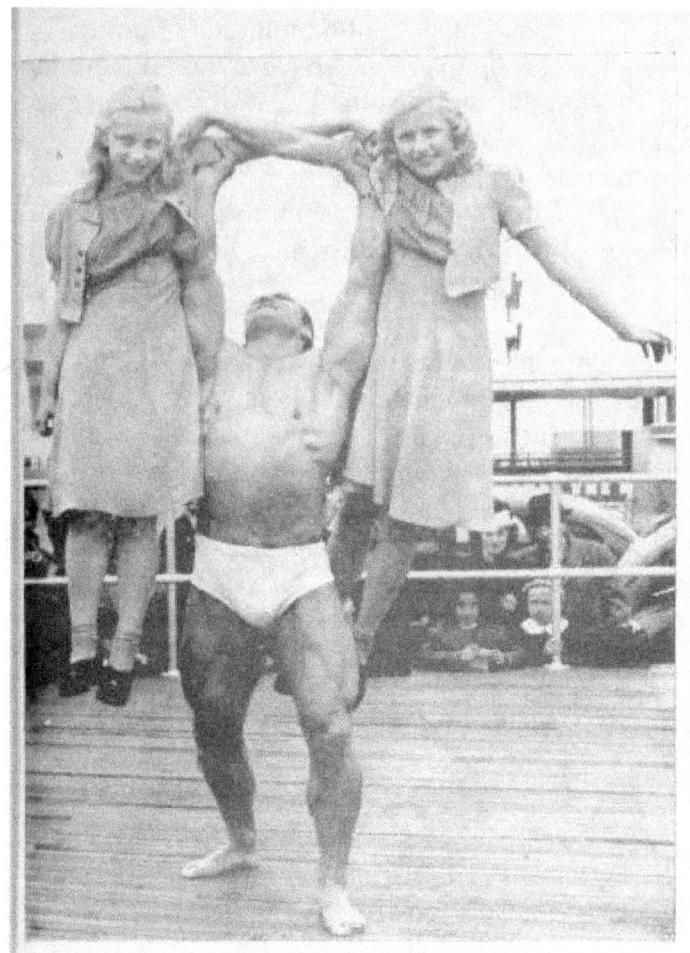

A press photo taken at the World's Fair in New York the morning after Grimek won the "Mr. America" title and was one of the place winners in the national weight-lifting championship. Grimek military pressed 285 in that contest and won five prizes in all. Here, at the request of the newspaper photographers, he is giving a moderate demonstration of his strength by lifting Anna and Mary Schusterich, blonde and attractive sisters of "Mr. New York"—Ludwig Schusterich of Brooklyn.

CHAPTER THREE
Inherited Physical Strength

An "authority" has written in his popular selling book, "If you don't want to be bald, castrate your grandfather." Impossible, of course, but he wishes to imply that profusion or absence of hair is solely the result of heredity. He tells us, too, that if we want to live long or be strong to select long-lived and powerful ancestors. It is true that our ancestors, in our own case heredity, do play an important part in determining the length of our lives, but how, we must wonder, did our parents, our grandparents and our great-greats manage to live so long? The lives of hard work and simplicity they lived make it possible for us to live longer and more fully. Similarly physical training and habits of right living will not only make it possible for us of today to live longer and more fully, but will bequeath in turn a longer life to our children and our children's children in the vast majority of cases.

The Bible tells us that the sins of the father will be experienced to the third and fourth generation. Similarly the careful living, the habits of eating, moderation in smoking or drinking, the strength and superhealth which are the result of proper exercise, progressive, heavy training, will improve the lives of generations to come three or four removed. By following the simple rules of living now, you are building up your strength and health bank account, preparing to leave a rich legacy to generations to come.

I have enumerated personal statistics concerning our young lifting champions of today. Some had poorer than a mediocre beginning. Others made the most of their heredity —trained fully the sound, vigorous and healthy body they inherited from their parents. Reaching the heights in strength and development will be easier for some than others. They have a better heredity, but no man need despair. It will require more effort, persistence, more years of training to be a superman if there is a poor beginning than if we are fortunate in being the offspring of superhealthy, strong ancestors; but persistence and proper training methods will get us there just the same. You can not determine in the beginning to which category you belong, whether it will require greater or lesser effort to attain your physical goals, but one thing sure, just as Longfellow said, "as sure as the vine grows round the stump," you'll attain your physical goals if you but make your start—follow proper progressive training methods and persist in your training.

There are unquestionably many men of gigantic strength who have inherited a large measure of their physical powers. Louis Cyr certainly inherited his vast body, huge bones and a fair share of his strength chiefly from his powerful mother. A contemporary, Horace Barre, a huge lethargic man by nature, who preferred not to extend himself, was another who inherited much of his strength. Many considered him to be as physically strong as Louis Cyr but he lacked the ability or the desire to extend himself. He walked across the gymnasium one day with a 1270 pound bar bell upon one shoulder.

When I was just a youngster I knew a very husky Y.M.C.A. physical director who had very powerful hands, wrists and forearms. He told me that his mother had extremely powerful hands and arms, unusual gripping power, enough power to make an average man wince with pain when she squeezed his hand. During my life I won many prizes at an event called canoe tilting. It is an aquatic imitation of the manner in which the knights of old fought with their horses and lances. One man sits on the bottom of the boat and paddles. The tilter stands with his feet upon the gunwales of the canoe; he is armed with a sixteen foot, vaulting, bamboo pole, on the end of which has been fastened a soccer football inflated to the limit and held in place with a canvas bag and a rubber socket.

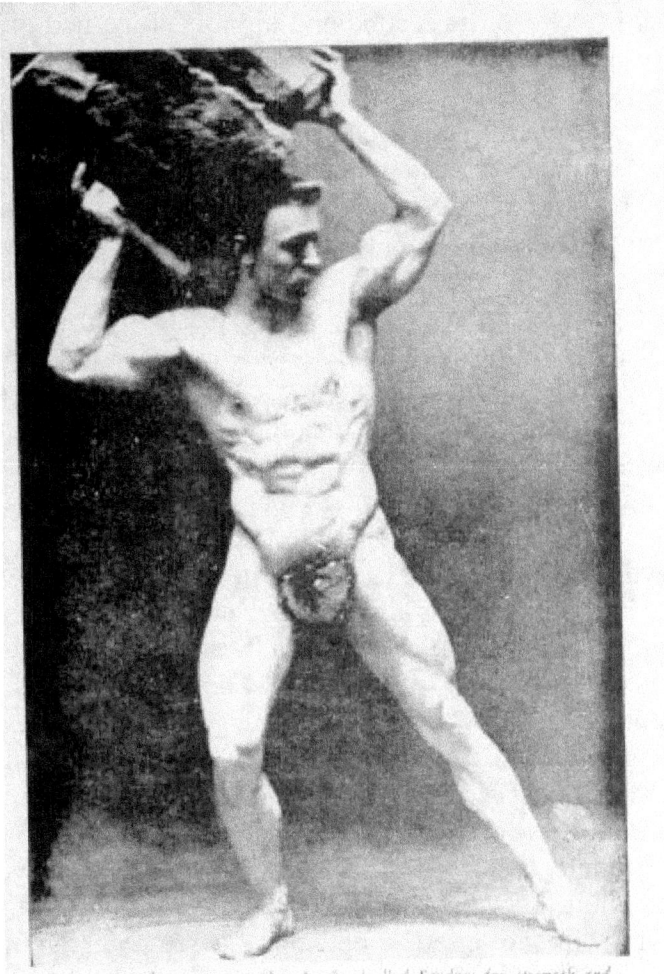

Bobby Pandour, a man who closely rivalled Sandow for strength and development, yet is little known as he was not as highly publicized as the great Sandow.

A very hard blow can be hit with this improvised weapon. The team who knocks the other tilter into the water, or upsets their boat, wins. I quickly found that the way to gain superiority was to develop the toes so that they could grasp the sides of the boat with a strength which would not permit them to be dislodged. I started lifting five pound dumbells between my second and big toes. I learned to pick up a twenty-five pound dumbell in this manner. Still later I developed the ability to chin myself under a small bridge lifting the seventy pound canoe meanwhile with my toes. As the newspapers said, "held on with the talons of an eagle," or "with a grip which must have come down to me from my forbears—my tree-climbing and tree-hanging ancestors, the monkeys." In fifteen years of canoe tilting competition I was never once forced off the gunwales and won many fine prizes and points for our club in this event. Was my ability acquired? Partly, for no one else used such a system. But my mother wears a nine triple A shoe, has the narrowest and the longest foot I have ever seen, with toes like fingers. So it's quite evident that I inherited a fair share of this ability. You will soon note that I am trying to prove that, while some of us have a more favorable heredity than others, if we do nothing about it we remain mediocre in our ability, while the man who is handicapped by nature yet persists in his training will reach the heights in the athletic or strength world. When I find a young man who gives unusual promise as a weight lifter I'll ask him questions: "Was your father strong?" "Yes," he'll reply, "the strongest man in our section." And I'll say, "Sorry, but you'll never get anywhere then. Your strength came too easy; you'll give up, quit, be satisfied. The man who reaches the top is the man with an inferior beginning who trains to make himself the equal of his more fortunate playmates." And there is considerable truth in what I tell these young fellows. There are exceptions to all rules, but few men become champions when well endowed by nature in the beginning. This was brought so forcefully to my attention in making the last trip to the Olympic Games. I was trainer for the

48

American weight lifting team and of course doing all I could to boost weight lifting on the entire trip. I became very well acquainted with the men from most teams, and I'll never cease to marvel at what a collection of cripples they were: men like Glen Cunningham, badly burned in a school fire as a child, informed that he would never walk again, who learned to run fast enough to defeat the world's best time after time, and to establish world's records; or " Hank " Dryer, whose arm as the result of a kiddy car accident when he was a child had grown crooked—badly distorted through improper setting—who had become the national hammer throwing champion; or Millard who had been frail and weak in the beginning, yet had developed himself to the point where he became the American wrestling champion at his weight and also the best wrestler in the world in his division; or Betty Robinson, who had been world's 100 meter champion at sixteen, severely injured at nineteen in an airplane accident, fractured skull, broken limbs, told that she would never run again, yet she became a member of the Olympic champion American relay team who won at Berlin. There were many others; physical training had made them the nation's best, and in many cases the world's best, in spite of their injuries or sadly deficient beginning.

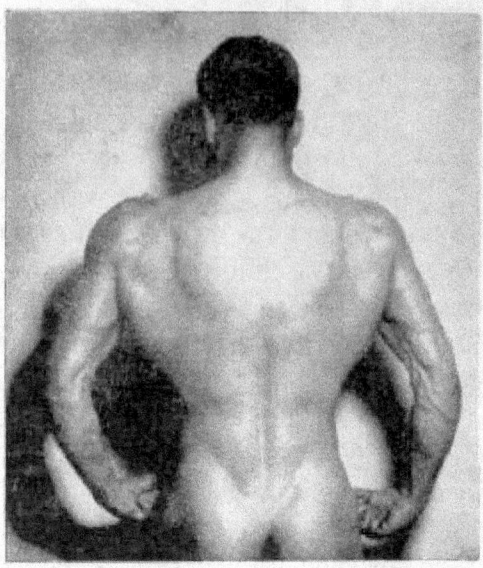

This powerful and shapely back belongs to Carl de Gloria of Mount Vernon, N. Y. Slender waist, wide-spreading latissimus, well-rounded deltoids, powerful spinae erector muscles make his physique an object of beauty to the admirer of the masculine physique.

I briefly mentioned in a previous chapter that Louis Uni, Apollon to the strength world, had married a tiny mite of a woman who dominated him completely, in turn nagging, arguing, coaxing him to make world's weight lifting history. But I failed to say that he came from a famous family of strong men, and that he was vastly stronger than either his parents or his grandparents—stronger than any man.

In this country we have our strong men and strong families too. Anyone who has read Strength and Health magazine, or others of my books, will remember a number of references to men of the name Nordquest, Joe and Adolph being the best known. They hail from Ashtabula, Ohio. The father of this famous family was tall and well made, but not markedly above the average in strength. The mother is rather small. I know six sons and one daughter to this union. I frequently hear from daughter Annie who, aside from being very proud of her famous brothers, had a just claim to the title of strong woman in her own right. She too was a strength performer early in her career.

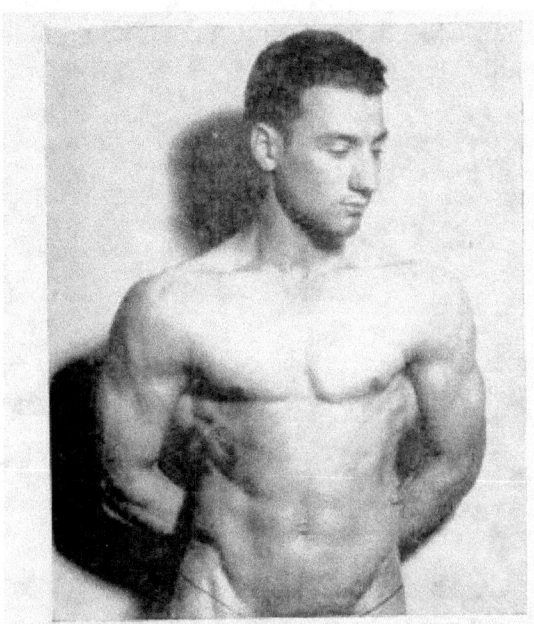

The other side of the young man on opposite page. While slender in general appearance, his well-developed pectoral muscles, sloping shoulders and columnar neck, with narrow waist and well-developed abdominals, create the effect much desired and admired by those who are training to acquire the Body Beautiful. Both photos by Lon of New York City.

Of the six sons, three of them are best known: Joe, Arthur, Adolph, veritable Vikings in build and truly marvels of muscular power. The other three sons had the same inherited qualities, were all naturally well built and much stronger than the average but none of them possesses the prodigious power or the magnificent proportions of his powerful brothers. They were born with the same inheritance, the same possibilities, and with proper training they no doubt would have attained physical power and excellence which would have placed them on a par with their brothers. They might have been just as remarkable as the three Nordquests all strength lovers remember so well. Joe,

Arthur and Adolph were enthusiastic devotees of athletics and strength, and trained with the sole idea of becoming supermen. All had the same opportunity, but the famous three voluntarily developed their possibilities and the power which has made them immortal. Their success was unquestionably due to inheritance, plus initiative—the will to be strong.

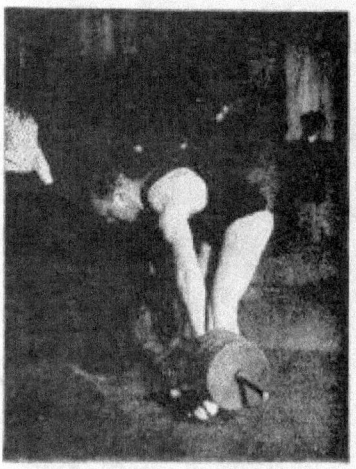
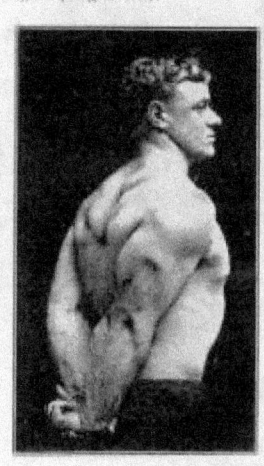

Left, Adolph Nordquest in 1916, setting his world's record in the stiff legged dead weight lift. He grasped the bar with knuckles front, and lifted 638 pounds to the height shown here. In the usual dead weight lifting style, the palms face each other, the legs are bent and the back is kept flat. This method requires great gripping power and back strength.

Right, Joe Nordquest at the age of 22 in 1916 at the time he bent pressed with the left hand the world's record poundage of 277¼ pounds. Although handicapped by a lower limb amputated as a result of a childhood accident, Joe Nordquest repeatedly set world's weight lifting records.

Many of the famous strong men of the past frankly admitted that a good share of their strength was inherited from one or both parents. Many of these men discovered in earliest boyhood that they were stronger than the average and from that beginning cultivated their strength to the point where they attained rank as "strong men" and are still known to devotees of strength throughout the world. In the early days of "train you by mail" physical instructors in this country a number of these men, notably Massimo, Pandour and even Sandow, were claimed by these training concerns as their pupils. We at times saw the splendid physique of Fred Rollon and these other powerful gentlemen gracing the advertisements of some other instructor, often a countryman who had a simple system of training which he offered for sale. It was misleading until a stop was put to it by organizations such as the Federal Trade Commission.

Some men acquire more than their share of strength in an easy manner. I know of many interesting cases of muscle men whose beautiful proportions and phenomenal strength are unquestionably due to their own efforts. Neither their father nor mother may be anything remarkable as physical specimens. Their brothers range from short and fat to tall and thin. These prominent athletes are usually taller than other members of their families because their enthusiasm for training at an early age has stimulated their growth. I have known these men who came from very ordinary parental stock to become so strong that they create amateur lifting records, and so beautifully shaped that they are winners at best-developed man contests, and are in demand as artists' or sculptors' models. These men were "exercise devotees" who worked for their physique while their very ordinary brothers were satisfied to muddle along with the strength and build they inherited.

I have written so long and enthusiastically concerning the men who have built their bodies from an ordinary beginning that I hope you are not getting the impression that I wish to minimize the value of a good inheritance. If you have parents who are fine, upstanding, and vigorous examples of manhood and womanhood, who have passed on to you these desirable physical attributes, then you will find it just that much easier to develop a body that is the last word in physical perfection. But you need not despair, on the other hand, if you have parents who are undersized, undeveloped or "just average"; with this less favorable beginning it will take you a little longer to become strong and well developed, require considerable more work, but you will become big and strong in time through persistent and intelligent effort.

Certain families are known for definite physical characteristics. These families run true to a particular type. You may know a family of Browns who are all quite tall, and a family of Smiths whose men are short and broad, and still another strain of humans in which slender, light-boned men will predominate. There are certain physical characteristics which persist in a particular strain for generation after generation. Two good examples of such characteristics are the Bourbon nose and the Hapsburg lip.

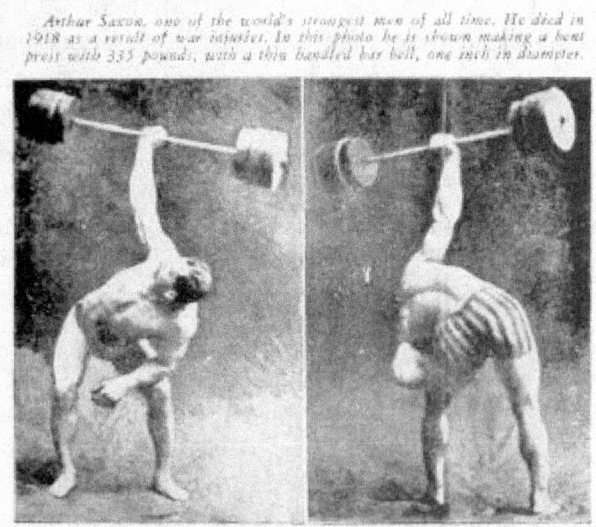

Arthur Saxon, one of the world's strongest men of all time. He died in 1918 as a result of war injuries. In this photo he is shown making a bent press with 335 pounds, with a thin handled bar bell, one inch in diameter.

There are so many erroneous ideas concerning physical development—many who believe that we are as we are, that we have nothing to do with improving our physical selves. If they see the picture of a strong man they will retort, "Aw, that guy was born that way." They believe that a man's physical self is in line with the Biblical query, "Can an Ethiopian change his skin or a leopard his spots?" They overlook the fact that there is a great difference between Ethiopians and leopards. The famous Queen of Sheba, who consorted with the even more famous King Solomon, was reported to be an Ethiopian. Ethiopians of today range in all colors from a hue no darker than an Arab to the blackest ebony. Some leopards have light spots, some dark ones, while others are black with hardly perceptible spots. There are of course inherited characteristics which cannot be changed. A colored man cannot turn himself into a white man, a Chinaman into an Indian, a blond Nordic into a natural brunette. Nor can a man change the size of his ears, the shape of his head nor the appearance of his nose unless he has an operation performed. These are all racial characteristics.

But the form, or the appearance, or the strength and size of an individual certainly can be altered. Men with light bones cannot expect as massive a development as the heavy boned man, but they can obtain a better proportioned development. While still in the growing stage the size of bones has been increased. There are a host of authentic reports of men who have increased their knee, wrist or hip size as a result of training. In one of my books, "Weight Lifting," I show a photo of myself endeavoring to wear the same coat I wore when I came home from France. Then it fitted loosely enough. I weighed at that time 180 pounds; now, at 265, I cannot come within a foot of closing the coat around my chest. This more than a foot of increase in chest girth took place after I had passed the age of twenty-one, when many people think that increased development is no longer possible. When your chest grows the shoulders must widen too; shoulders can be widened and chest enlarged until a man is at least fifty years of age. They will grow more rapidly in his young manhood, but they will grow when middle age is reached. Part of the growth is in muscle development, but there is a spreading of the shoulder blades or clavicles, a thickening and lengthening of the tendons and attachments which first of all makes the body framework wider. With the addition of two or three inches in width due to a thickening of the deltoid muscles of the shoulders it is not difficult to see how a man's shoulders can become a great deal broader. Naturally when the shoulders broaden, the chest enlarges, becomes rounder and deeper; a man is bigger all over as his bodyweight and muscular development have increased to keep pace with the shoulders and chest.

Hereditary physical characteristics persist only when for generation after generation the males of the same family remain in the same environment and continue with the same employment. Physical activity at an early age stimulates rapid growth. Therefore should the sons of an undersized bookkeeper, whose ancestors for generations have been office workers, be placed at hard outdoor work in earliest youth, they will grow much larger and stronger than their parents or brothers and sisters who continue at light work. Similarly the young man who early in life determines to build his body through progressive weight training will grow much more rapidly and end by being far bigger, heavier and stronger than his father and other male relatives. If the sons of powerful woodsmen or farmers would be removed from their parents' environment at birth, be reared and later employed in the city for at least the first or second generation, they would be stronger and larger than the average, but not quite as large or strong as father or brothers who continued at the parents' former mode of living.

Many writers discussing inherited characteristics have endeavored to prove that heredity, and heredity only, deter-

mines the type of man we are to be. They cite the cases of
many professional strong men of the past, some of whom
had powerful parents, so it would seem that their arguments
are based on considerable logic. One writer informs us that
Shakespeare inherited unusual physical strength, possessed
spendidly shaped legs, and had based his opinion entirely
on a recent and ideological statue of the bard of Avon. All
history points to the fact that Shakespeare was a small and
slight man.

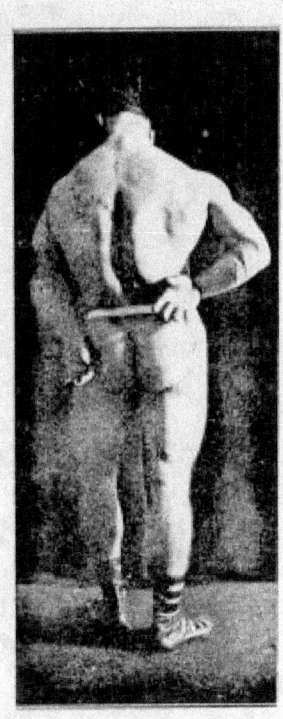

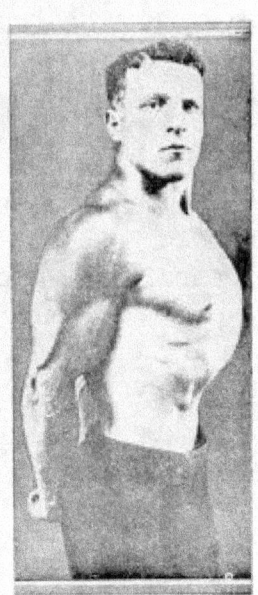

Below, Henry Steinborn, long
famous as the strongest man in
wrestling, as he appeared in
1920, when he arrived upon
these shores to set world's
weight lifting records. Excelling
in the quick lifts, it is said that
he cleaned and jerked 375
pounds when the bar which
should have weighed 350 was
overloaded. On this occasion he
exceeded Louis Cyr's record of
347 pounds.

Above, Tony Massimo, one of
the most muscular men the world
has ever seen. In this photo he is
5' 8" in height, has a 17-inch neck,
16½-inch upper arm, 13-inch forearm, 47-inch chest, 30-inch waist,
and weighs 200 pounds.

One writer endeavored to prove his point that inherited strength counts most by telling us that Henry Ward Beecher was a man of imposing physique and great strength. He quoted Beecher himself to show that his size, development and strength were largely inherited. Mr. Beecher related that his father was so strong that he could lift a four hundred pound barrel of cider a couple of feet from the ground; and that his grandfather could lift the same barrel overhead and drink from the bunghole while holding it there. Beecher hailed from New England; his ancestors for long years had been farm folks, and in his earlier years he himself had been a farmer before he became a preacher. The vigorous outdoor work at which he spent all of his time in earlier youth, and the forceful life he led as a frontier preacher helped him develop the great strength for which he was famed. He inherited the physical vigor, the healthy body, but not his ancestors' gigantic strength. It is undeniable that all of us inherit some possibility of strength. The Beecher case could easily be reversed. A small, undersized, physically weak factory worker, who had spent his life from childhood working twelve hours daily in a poorly ventilated mill or factory, might move to the country and there become the father of big upstanding children who would in turn be the parents of still larger, stronger children. Thus environment, the life the children led, would be of greater importance than the poor physical inheritance with which they made a beginning. Recently published statistics show that in Great Britain as well as in this country the average farm worker is a couple of inches taller and five to ten pounds heavier than the average city worker. More fresh air, fresh food and considerable muscular work have made the farm hand bigger and taller than the city dweller. Those who claim that physical strength can be had in no way except by inheritance are continually being confronted with cases which disprove their theories. You may have heard a young man say, "Yes, I am pretty strong, but you ought to see my father; he is twice my age and twice as strong as I am." If the father overhears this remark, he will laugh and say, "That may all be true because Harry never had to perform the hard work I had to when I was a boy."

I have already cited the cases of a number of young strength champions who had a favorable heredity, but they attained the physical heights through training. I could tell you of hundreds of additional young men who early in life became interested in physical training who are a great deal larger and stronger than their fathers. The fathers frequently went in for business, the professions or sedentary work of some sort and did not develop their own physical possibilities. A few years ago athletics were unpopular and systematic exercise considered to be a waste of time by the majority of people. They thought that the exercise devotee was a show-off, training only to put big muscles on the out- side of his body. They were not cognizant of the fact that the development of muscle is secondary in progressive physical training. The way we feel is most important and this comes about through an improvement of the internal processes and the strengthening of the organs on which our lives depend. Increased circulation, improved respiration, better appetite, better digestion, perfect elimination are only a few of the internal improvements which are the result of exercise. But this was not so well understood in our fathers' day, and many of them failed to grow as large or strong as they would have done had physical training been as popular as it is today. One thing sure, we are producing in this country a superior race of men, men who will be larger and stronger with each additional generation as long as they continue with simple living and exercise.

When I briefly mention the fact that I feel younger than I did twenty years ago, that I have so much pep and energy that if I felt any better I would have to take something, that

I haven't had a headache or a sick stomach for thirty years, that I never experience the slightest physical irregularity, haven't taken a physic since childhood, people say, "You're lucky. You must have inherited a fine body." I won't dispute the fact that my parents were normal and healthy; more and more with each passing day I appreciate the physical normalcy with which they endowed me, but I am the only one of the brothers or sister in the immediate family, cousins or aunts or uncles, who never has physical complaints. My mother never ceases to be astonished that my letters are always cheerful; never a word about aches, pains, sicknesses or ills, while letters from others have little to tell except that Mary was sick for a few days, Bill has a severe cold, Helen has a headache, John has rheumatism. No, it isn't luck or heredity that makes me the leading contender for the title of "world's healthiest man." It's the life I lead. Twenty-five years ago I graduated from high school; since then I have been so unbelievably busy it hardly seems possible. I finished the season of 1926 as a member of a national champion eight oar rowing crew. That fall I was married, was working intensively, trying to make a success of the business in which I was engaged, obtained very little sleep, and became so tired that I fell asleep on my feet while working at the county fair, fell into a puddle of water and lay there asleep. I continued to work that way all the next year. Yet somehow I managed to win the national A.A.U. weight lifting championship, the boxing championship, the wrestling championship, the hand ball championship, the hexathlon championship, win victories in boat racing, swim on the Y.M.C.A. swimming team, breast stroke being my strongest point, run on the mile relay team, put the shot and win the county quoit pitching championship. That year is just one example of the way I have driven myself all these years. In the last few years I have written over a thousand magazine articles; this year, with all the angles of the business in which I engage, writing thousands of letters, a book every two months, and as we publish the books and I read every one of them eight times it takes a lot of work; travel a great deal yet find time enough to train a bit and improve physically with each passing year. I work at least sixteen hours a day—just the sort of activity that makes a man old before his time, brings him to mental or physical collapse, but I get better and better. I feel like a million. So it isn't heredity but right living and exercise which make the difference. And exercise is what will make the difference in your case too.

I must mention myself at times for I think that my own case is one of the best arguments I know against the inherited strength theory. I positively, definitely and emphatically know that my present strength and health are the result not of heredity but of my own constant, intensive efforts at self-improvement.

There are men, I must repeat again, who are like the huge draft horse and the bulldog, who have inherited a great measure of strength. Henry Steinborn, Arthur Saxon, Louis Cyr, Louis Uni, best known as Apollon, George Hackenschmidt, the present world's lifting champion, Joseph Manger, all undoubtedly inherited more than average strength. But they made the most of it through training, or their names would not be bywords in the strength world. Arthur Saxon and George Hackenschmidt both have said that in boyhood they were always much stronger than their playmates. Louis Cyr at fifteen was stronger than two ordinary strong men. Louis Uni was a professional strong man at the same youthful age and was far stronger than other mature men. But his strength did constantly increase through physical training and he became much stronger than his father or grandfather who had been professional strong men before him.

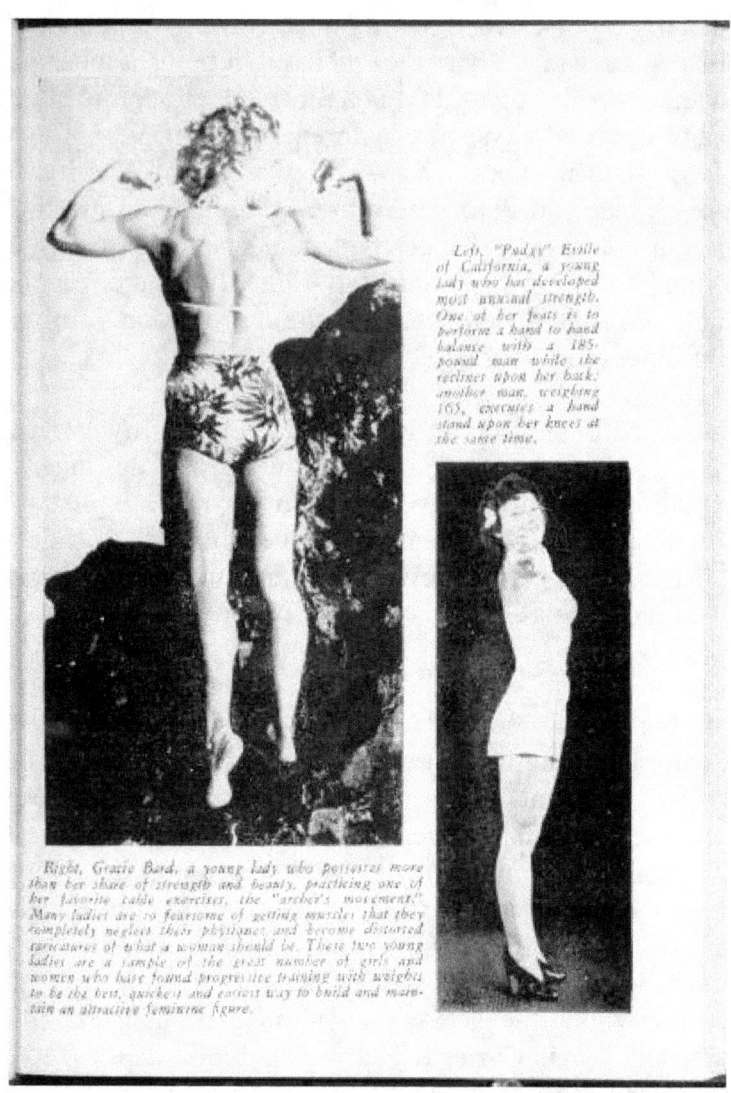

Right, Gracie Bard, a young lady who possesses more than her share of strength and beauty, practicing one of her favorite table exercises, the "archer's movement." Many ladies are so fearsome of getting muscles that they completely neglect their physiques and become distorted caricatures of what a woman should be. These two young ladies are a sample of the great number of girls and women who have found progressive training with weights to be the best, quickest and easiest way to build and maintain an attractive feminine figure.

Many people believe that Sandow was the strongest man of his time. He was very strong, one of the strongest for his weight, but there were many men of his time who were stronger than he. He is most famed for his extraordinary physique, a physique which improved with each passing year, until he attained perfection at fifty-eight, which I believe has never been equalled. When he was young he was quite average in size, and, as he wrote, he was a "mere stripling"; the bar bell and the dumbell built his great physique and strength. A great many other strong men make the same statement. I have already mentioned some of today's champions who started with a very ordinary development and reached championship heights. There are a great many more well-known men of might and muscle who had similar experiences. Eddie Harrison and Bob Mitchell are two who became national champion lifters, both of whom weighed just over a hundred pounds when they were in high school. Gord Venables had tried many forms of athletics and weighed just one hundred and fifty-four pounds when he started weight lifting. He became a powerful, beautifully built two hundred pounder, a better all- around athlete and a man who never fails to place in national or North American weight lifting competition. Of the old timers, Kenneth Terril, Bobby Pandour and Antone Matysek are three famous men of muscle who had a very frail beginning, but developed to the point where they are nearly immortal for their strength and proportions. Thomas Inch of England, a famous old timer who built himself from a lightweight to a heavyweight champion; Ronald Walker, a tall undeveloped youth, who became British champion and world's record holder; or Al Manger of the nearby city of Baltimore who actually did weigh ninety- seven pounds when past the age of twenty-one, who increased his weight to one hundred and ninety pounds and won three consecutive national weight lifting titles and became a member of the 1932 Olympic team, are others whose success came as the result of training rather than heredity.

So many men have succeeded from a very ordinary beginning it must be convincing to you that you, too, can transform yourself into a physical marvel if you will work hard, persistently and intelligently, to gain that end. You may be discouraged at times when you find fellows who seem to inherit strength, to have more naturally than you have after months or years of work.

There are young fellows who carelessly display a sixteen-inch arm which they obtained from very little exercise while others work a lifetime and don't attain such a sizeable arm.

It is discouraging if you are not numbered among the fortunate ones who have inherited strength and development. But make the best of it; it will take you longer to gain your desired end but you'll ultimately surpass the other person. It's sort of a case of the tortoise and the hare. Everyone knew that the hare could run rings around a tortoise; it did, then lay down to sleep while the tortoise kept toiling on toward the end of the race and victory. Similarly the person who gains rapidly doesn't value his gains and too often ceases to exercise while the persistent physical culturist continues and surpasses him in time.

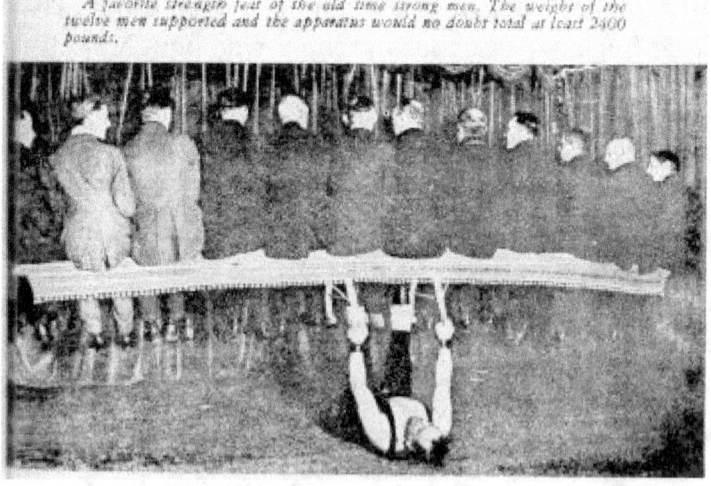

A favorite strength feat of the old time strong men. The weight of the twelve men supported and the apparatus would no doubt total at least 2400 pounds.

These fortunate fellows who inherit more than their share of strength and development more often than not are like the son who has inherited wealth from his father. He has never had to count pennies, to work long hours for it, to scheme and contrive means to make money, and rarely appreciates the value of money. Few strong men have sons who rival them in strength and development because their sons seldom realize the value of their natural advantages, and almost never take the trouble to improve or cultivate them. I cannot recall the name of any strong man who has sons of equal strength.

These fortunate people who inherit a good measure of strength are reluctant to perform the hard kind of work; by work I mean heavy exercise, which produces extraordinary world-beating strength. As they have never been weak they have never experienced the full craving for strength. Just as the son of a captain of industry who has never been hungry or cold, never so completely out of money that the bill collectors were chasing him, will never plan and strive and work unendingly to amass a fortune such as his father did.

In our modern world respect is accorded to the "self-made man," to a man who has attained his position entirely through his own energy, ability and initiative. More people understand and appreciate success as measured in position and dollars, but fortunately an increasing number have come to acquire similar respect for the man who, starting with a frail, weak body, builds himself until he is a model of manly strength and symmetry. He has shoulders which are broad because he made them broad, a powerful back because he made it that way, has not only made himself stronger and superbly built all over but has literally made himself over. There have been men who were prone to glorify the strong man who inherited his strength "and sneer or make fun of the made strong man, yet it seems to me that the man who reached the heights of strength and development from a poor beginning deserves more credit for achieving this success through his own efforts.

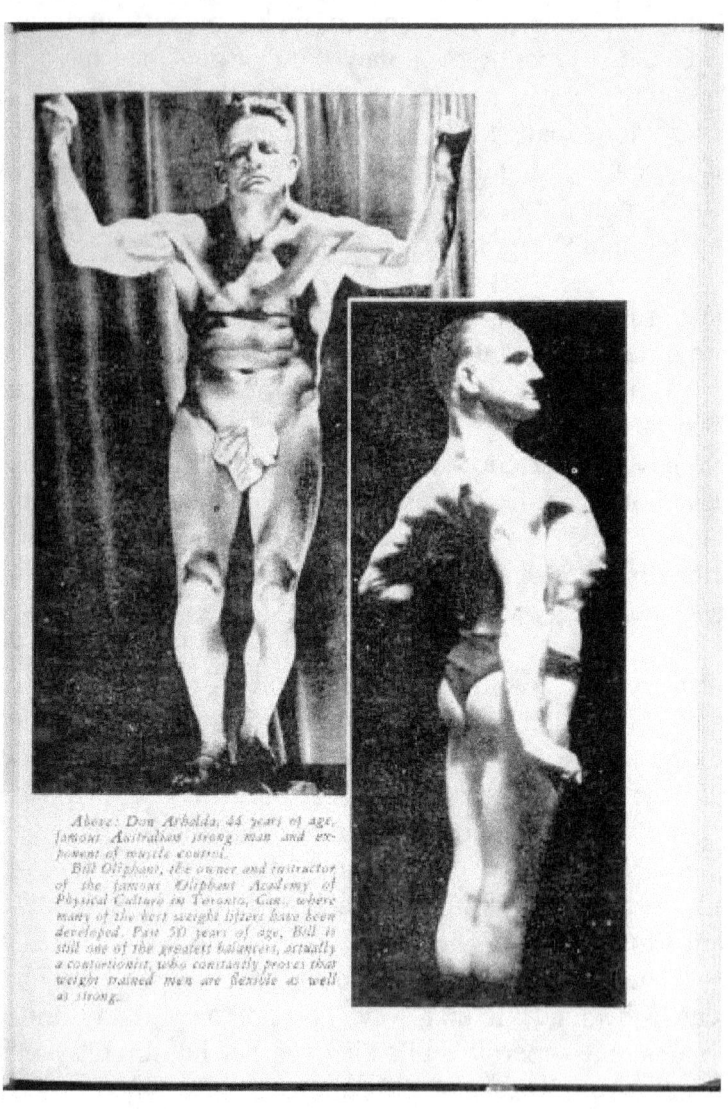

Above: Don Arbolda, 44 years of age, famous Australian strong man and exponent of muscle control.

Bill Oliphant, the owner and instructor of the famous Oliphant Academy of Physical Culture in Toronto, Can., where many of the best weight lifters have been developed. Past 50 years of age, Bill is still one of the greatest balancers, actually a contortionist, who constantly proves that weight trained men are flexible as well as strong.

CHAPTER FOUR
Bone Size in Regard to Strength

A draft horse has tremendously heavy bones which are thick through their entire length and from end to end. A race horse may stand as tall as the draft horse but has much lighter bones and less weight. This difference in construction is the true mark of heredity, the result of selective breeding for many generations. The heavily-muscled bulldog and the greyhound offer us the same contrast. The young draft horse with no effort on its part grows heavy and powerful as does the bulldog even though it may lead the most indolent of lives.

These well-known characteristics of animals might cause the light-boned man at first thought to despair of ever being able to develop strength and muscle. He might say, "What's the use? All my people are tall and slender, with- out noticeable development. I can't do anything about it." And right across the street from this light-boned man, if he lives in the city, or on the next farm, if he lives in the country, might be a family whose male members are heavy-boned, deep-chested, broad-shouldered, and who are the possessors of heavy limbs, chiefly the result of heredity.

Many people believe that slender wrists and ankles are proof of an aristocratic ancestry, while heavy ankles, wrists and bones are a sign that one's ancestors have been peasants, or at least have lived lives of hard work. It is proof if you inherit big ankles and wrists, large bones and broad shoulders, that some of your immediate ancestors have done hard work, at least during the last several generations. Slender wrists and ankles in a woman add to her attractiveness and make it easy for her to obtain beautiful proportions, but there is no reason why a man should prefer these slender effeminate joints.

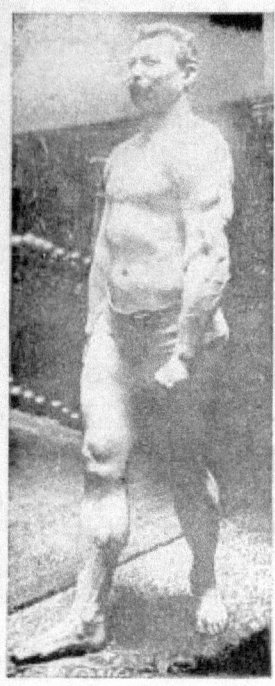

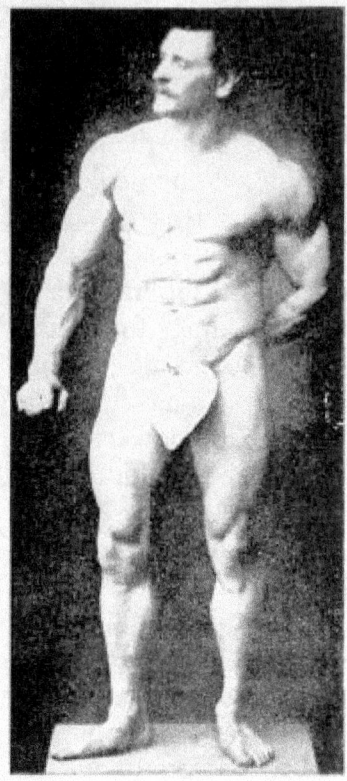

One of the best photos of Eugene Sandow.

In taking stock of yourself in an endeavor to determine just what you may expect in the way of development, measurement of the wrists, ankles, hips and shoulders will give you a good idea of the size of your bones. When you see a tall young man with big hips, and big hands and feet, you feel sure that there is a young man who is destined to be a really big powerful man when his body fills out to fit his extremities. But sometimes the hands and feet only seem large because of the relative undevelopment of other parts of the body. Certainly when there is a big wrist, knees

68

and ankles, there is more foundation on which to build. Greater muscular bulk is more easily obtained, but it is just as hard to develop perfect measurements, for the muscles must become very large in proportion.

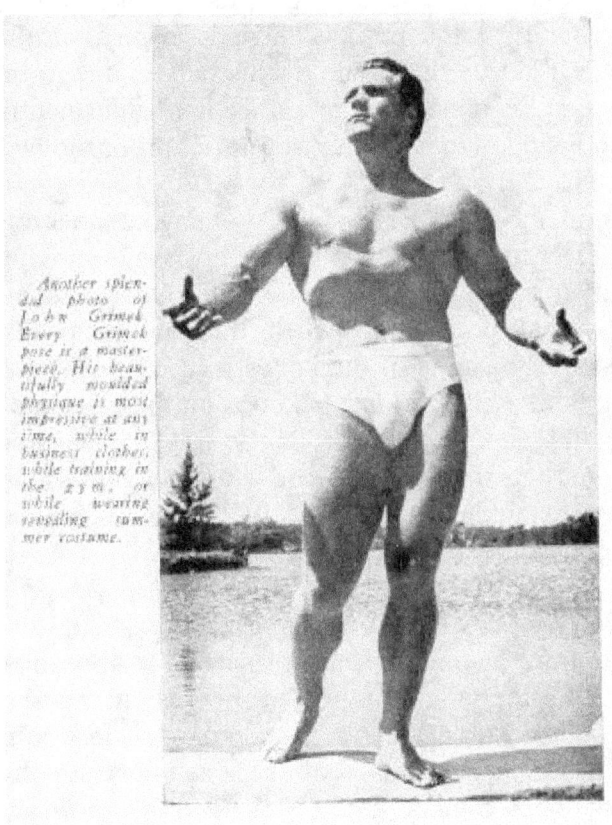

Another splendid photo of John Grimek. Every Grimek pose is a masterpiece. His beautifully moulded physique is most impressive at any time, while in business clothes, while training in the gym, or while wearing revealing summer costume.

John Grimek has a most unusual size to his wrist; part of this is due to the terrific development of the ligaments and tendons, but the bones are of tremendous size, as is evidenced by the protuberance at the wrist. While there are some men who have scarcely a noticeable bone at the thumb side of the wrist and only a small knob at the little finger side, John Grimek has tremendous lumps there, showing that his bone is huge. Similarly he has big elbows, ankles and knees, but he has developed such unusual musculature that his joints are small in comparison. His hips are very sturdy and of good size, as Grimek is one of the strongest men in the world, in spite of the fact that he usually weighs less than 200 pounds. He has tremendous muscular bulk at the points where it is most useful and attractive. It is true that some of this bulk is due to the size and shape of his bones, but he trained hard and scientifically to mould his body to its present beautiful proportions.

If you remember your physiology and your anatomy you will recollect that the bones of the limbs are long with large knobs upon the ends. The shape of the knobs varies with the individual bones and when the knobs are big the thickness of the shafts of the bones is also large. Of course the thick bone will have larger knobs on the ends and when there are larger knobs which can be felt or measured it is evident that the shaft of the bone is also large. A man with larger wrists, ankles, and elbows will have correspondingly larger bone shafts.

All muscles taper off into bones, every tendon fastens to a muscular fibre at one end and to a bone at the other end. There is considerable variation in the design and shape of these tendons; some are thick and round, some long and thin, others flat. A number of these tendons are fastened well down upon the bone, others close to the knob, and still others work through grooves in the bone; as definite places have been moulded in each bone for the passage of these tendons, it is evident that there are larger openings on a bigger bone and also that the tendons which fill these grooves must be bigger. With this thought in mind it is reasonable to arrive at the conclusion that with bigger joints there are bigger bones; with bigger bones, bigger tendons; and with bigger tendons there should be bigger muscles.

When big joints with the resulting size in all other parts are an inherited characteristic, it may seem discouraging to the individual who has smaller bones and smaller attachments to hope to obtain a development which compares even favorably with the bigger boned man. This latter type of person procures a well-developed body so much easier. While the light-boned man may train for years to obtain a fifteen-inch arm, the heavy-boned man obtains this size of arm so easily that he does not value it.

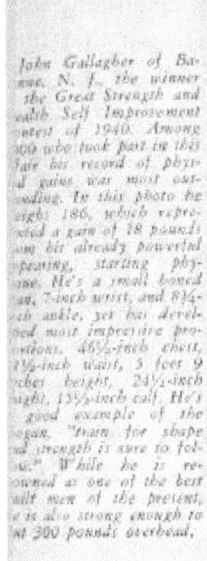
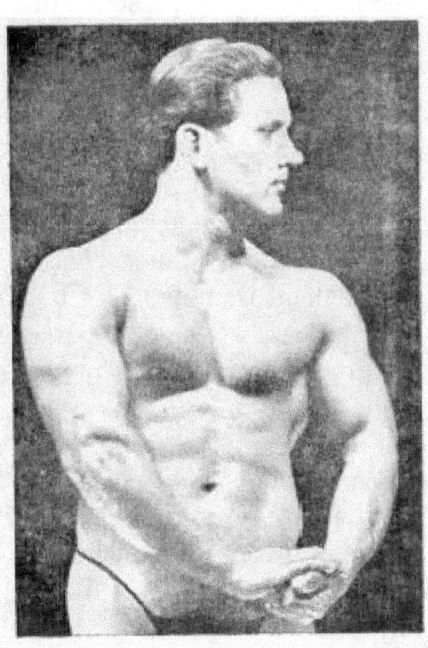

John Gallagher of Barre, N. J., the winner the Great Strength and Health Self Improvement contest of 1940. Among 300 who took part in this fair his record of physical gains was most outstanding. In this photo he weighs 186, which represented a gain of 18 pounds on his already powerful physique, starting physique. He's a small boned man, 7-inch wrist, and 8½-inch ankle, yet has developed most impressive proportions. 46½-inch chest, 8½-inch waist, 5 feet 9 inches height, 24½-inch thighs, 15½-inch calf. He's a good example of the slogan, "train for shape and strength is sure to follow." While he is renowned as one of the best built men of the present, he is also strong enough to put 300 pounds overhead.

In a group such as we have here in York, including many of the world's strongest and best-built men, we have men of all types. One of these, a man who is famed for his strength, development, lifting and all-around athletic ability, is Gord Venables. Gord has small arms in proportion to the really fine breadth of shoulders he possesses, but his arm, which is much smaller than other champions of his weight, looks

71

attractive, well moulded or well developed because his joints are small; and his broad shoulders and fine limbs look even better because he has narrow hips, small for a two hundred pounder such as he is at present.

The idea that I will continue to write about in this chapter is that natural advantages are a great help—they speed the acquisition of strength and development; but the man who does not have these natural advantages to begin with need not despair, for the annals of the world of strength and development, past and present, offer a great many illustrations of men who have apparent disadvantages, yet have reached the heights. Many men believe that they are naturally in the draft horse or race horse class and feel that nothing they can do will overcome this condition appreciably. But the fact is that all humans are of such mixed ancestry that there is never the great divergence of types which is found with animals. There is a variance in the height and skeletal framework of humans but not nearly as much as in the case of the five pound miniature Doberman Pinscher (terrier) and the 181 pound great Dane we have here.

Although small bones are a hindrance in obtaining muscular size, they are not a preventative in acquiring splendid proportions and great strength, for the bones do not control the development of the bulk or the belly of the muscle, and the small joints with a beautifully developed muscular body are things of beauty to behold. Countless men have developed splendid muscular proportions in spite of small bones. In my years of teaching body-building methods designed to produce the physical desires of those who follow my methods, I have received well over 10,000 testimonials from those who enthusiastically extol the results they have obtained. Many hundreds of these letters with measurements have been published in Strength and Health magazine. Each month there are a good number of them. They attest better than any other proof the results which can be had.

So many writers of these letters have gained ten to twenty pounds, or even more, in a period of three months; their chests have deepened and increased in circumference; their shoulders have broadened and thickened; limbs became so much larger and more powerful. These men were, in the beginning, of all ages, shapes and conditions, and had varying physical desires. All who persist—first aspire and then perspire—have made remarkable physical improvement. If they had not believed that they could improve, if they had not been convinced by the results others had obtained, most of them would not have attained the proportions, the strength and development they now possess.

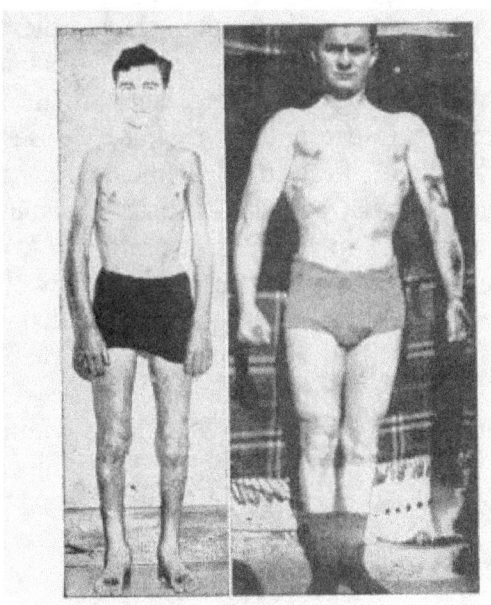

An extraordinary "before and after" case, W. A. Arnold of Wellington, N. Z. There is a little more than two years between these photos, the first taken January 30, 1936, and the second August 13, 1938. The two years of barbell training wrought an amazing change and improvement.

Each year about April, or perhaps a bit earlier—in March—there are a great many people after a long cold winter who begin to ponder about the pleasures the summer season offers. They think of their vacations and the fun they would like to have this summer—fun they didn't have last summer because they were ashamed of their bodies. But during this winter they learned of Strength and Health magazine, read some of the Success Stories each issue contains, and decided that they would do something about it. The young man follows the advice given in one of the articles he has read, takes a physical inventory of himself, stands in front of the mirror and looks himself over. He stretches out the arms first of all, for most men believe that arm strength and development are proof of bodily strength. Looking at his arms they seem so thin and undeveloped that he might despair of ever doing anything with them if he were not made of stern enough stuff that he is willing to start and persist in his methods. He flexes the arm and there is hardly a change in the position of the muscles— no change in the back of the arm; a slight swelling curve in the biceps or front of the arm. So different from what he observes in the great development of the arm of Grimek, who, aside from the Mr. America title and the Most Muscular Man in America, title, also won the Best-Developed Arm title. In the Grimek arm, when flexed, there is a great swelling curve to the lower arm; a huge thick and powerful hump to the upper arm. But turn that picture around (his picture on the August, 1940, cover of Strength and Health we refer to now) and note that amazing forearm. Why, the swelling of the muscles in that forearm looks like the upper arm of most champion lifters.

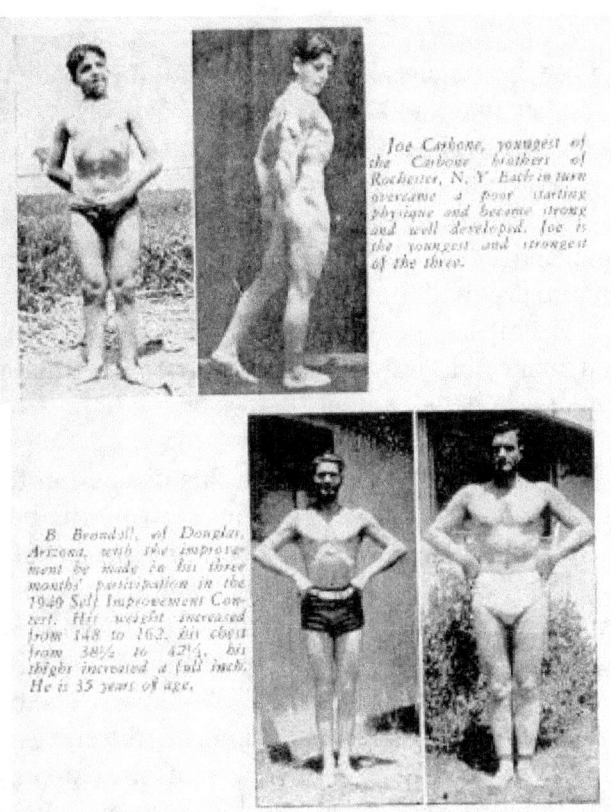

Joe Carbone, youngest of the Carbone brothers of Rochester, N. Y. Each in turn overcame a poor starting physique and became strong and well developed. Joe is the youngest and strongest of the three.

B. Brendall, of Douglas, Arizona, with the improvement he made in his three months' participation in the 1940 Self Improvement Contest. His weight increased from 148 to 162, his chest from 38½ to 42¼, his thigh increased a full inch. He is 35 years of age.

The beginner takes out the tape and finds that he has an upper arm of just eleven and a half inches, a wrist like an undeveloped girl's. But he persists. The weeks and months roll by, three months of them, and he has put on some weight and muscle—fourteen pounds of weight and two and a half inches on his biceps; fourteen inches—not large compared to the eighteen-inch arms of Grimek and Stanko, the seventeen-inch arm of Zagurski, the sixteen-inch arm of Terlazzo or Elmer Farnham, but a gain nevertheless. With that gain he is no longer ashamed that his arm be seen and he looks forward to receiving some compliments for having improved his arm so much. A fourteen-inch arm on a young man so slender is a really fine arm.

But suppose he persists, trains regularly for another year, makes another two and a half inches of gain. Now he truly has something, a sixteen-and-a-half-inch arm with a wrist of only seven inches. And this imaginary case I am citing is quite possible: two and a half inches in three months, another two and a half inches in the next year of training. After that there will be gains but they will come much slower, and will be accompanied with a shapeliness which will soon make this light-boned man acclaimed nationally for his great arm development.

I am writing most about the arms in this discussion for they are best understood, and chiefly thought of by the beginner in physical training. What I write about the arms is also true of the legs and other parts of the body. Most persons only consider their wrists when they believe they can or cannot obtain good-sized arms. In the upper arm there is but one bone, but in the lower arm there are two bones. The bone of the upper arm is known as the humerus, the lower as the radius and the ulna. The two bones of the forearm run roughly parallel to each other and the shape and position of these bones control to a great extent the shape and size of the forearm. If these bones are so constructed that they lie close together the forearm will be rather narrow when you hold the arm out in front of you with the palm up, unless of course you are an old hand at physical training and have developed considerable muscle on your forearm—then you have already overcome any unfavorable starting condition. But if there is a considerable space between these forearm bones, the forearm will be broad and you are already on the road to having a nicely developed arm.

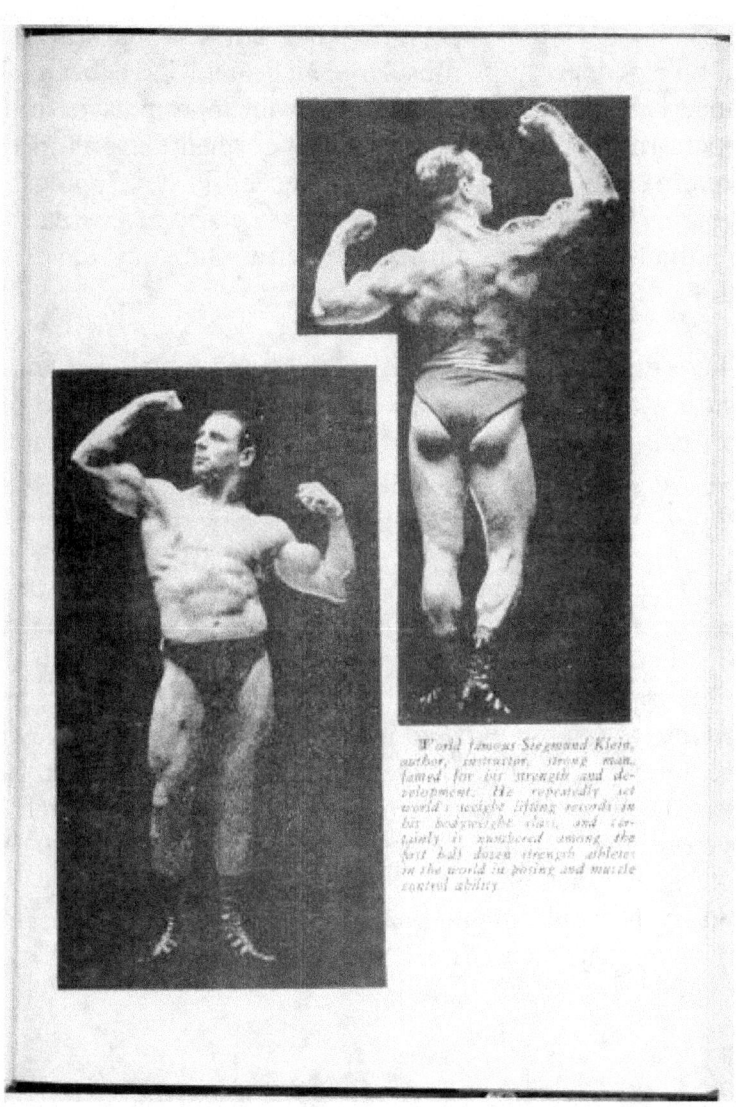

World famous Siegmund Klein, author, instructor, strong man, famed for his strength and development. He repeatedly set world's weight lifting records in his bodyweight class, and certainly is numbered among the first half dozen strength athletes in the world in posing and muscle control ability.

The forearm bones have knobs on their ends and if there is a big knob this alone will have a tendency to set them well apart, making the wrist bigger and the forearm broader to begin with. Small bones can set a definite limit to the size which will ultimately be acquired in the lower arm, but the single bone of the upper arm does not set this limit and really big upper arm muscles can be and have been obtained by light-boned men. There is far more muscle in the upper arm in relation to the bone size than there is in the forearm. Many men have not succeeded in developing big forearms in spite of intensive efforts because of this narrow and light-boned effect in the forearm. But they have developed splendid upper arms.

I have given a great deal of thought and have done much figuring and research work to determine the proportions that can be obtained with certain bone or joint measurements. In my book, "Big Arms," and how to develop them, I supplied the measurements of many of the nation's biggest-armed men. I have used the tape a great deal on other men's arms and have failed to find an arm in which the forearm has been twice as large as the wrist— that is, with the forearm held straight, merely tensed or with the wrist turned in slightly. With the forearm flexed a man like Grimek, with a big wrist, at least eight inches, and a sixteen-inch forearm, would have double the size of his wrists. But even the amazing development of his forearm, which is fourteen and a quarter inches straight as compared to his eight-inch wrist, is just 1.82 times the size of the wrist. And it is doubtful if there is a better-developed arm anywhere than John Grimek's.

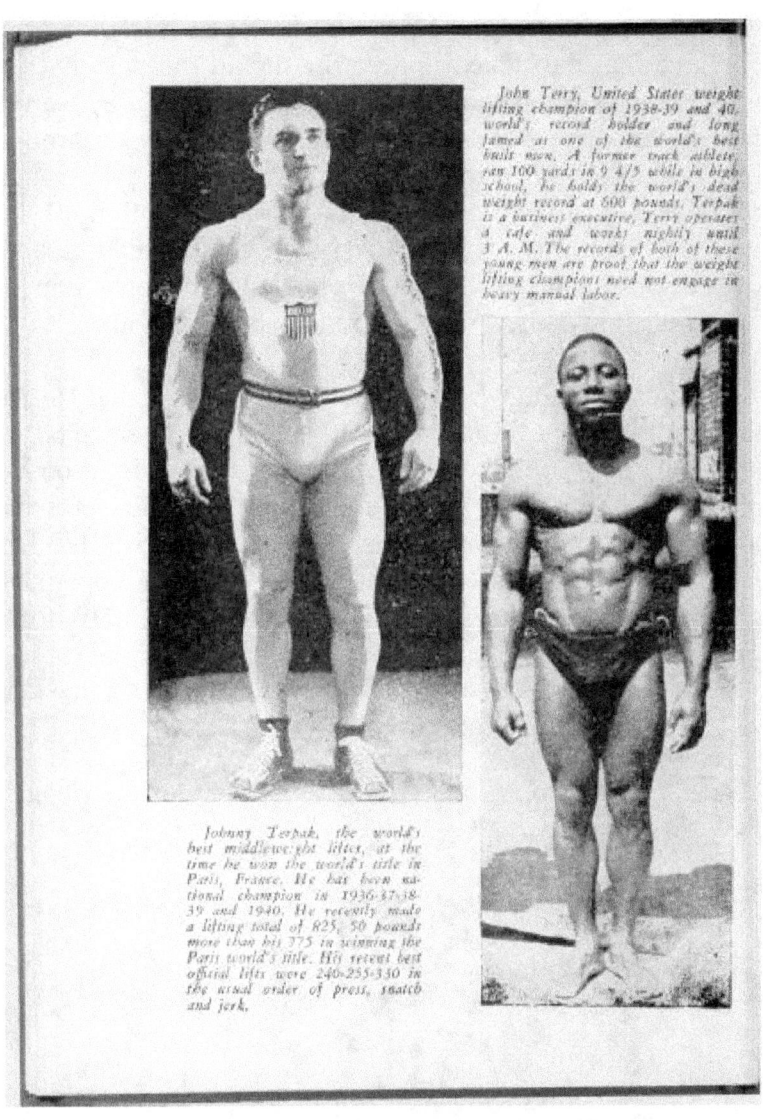

I believe the ultimate in development that an average man could expect would be a forearm 1.90 times the size of the wrist. Grimek's upper arm when held in what we term the No. 2 position, with the upper arm flexed to its limit, and the clenched fist near the shoulder, measures 17.5 inches.

This would be twenty-one per cent larger than the forearm. I believe that the flexed upper arm should measure twenty per cent more than the lower arm; for instance, a twelve-inch lower arm, a fourteen-and-a-half-inch upper arm; a thirteen-inch lower arm, an upper arm of 15.6; a 13.5 inch lower arm, an upper arm of 16.20. From these figures you will note that a man with a seven-inch wrist should be able to develop a forearm of 13.3 inches and an upper arm of sixteen inches. This would be a really splendid arm.

John Gallagher, the winner of the Great Strength and Health Self-Improvement Contest of 1940, a contest in which 6,000 ambitious body builders officially entered, is a light-boned man who has gained nearly ideal and very im- pressive proportions. Starting with a seven-inch wrist he has developed an impressive-appearing and powerful upper arm which measures sixteen and five-eighths inches. His fore-arm of thirteen inches is 1.87 per cent larger than the wrist.

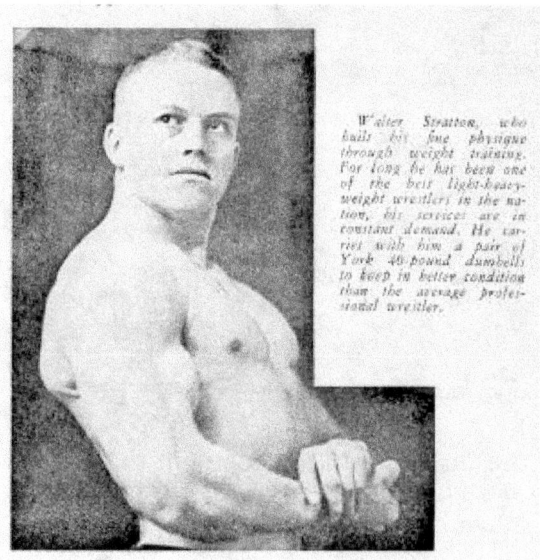

Walter Stratton, who built his fine physique through weight training. For long he has been one of the best light-heavyweight wrestlers in the nation, his services are in constant demand. He carries with him a pair of York 40-pound dumbells to keep in better condition than the average professional wrestler.

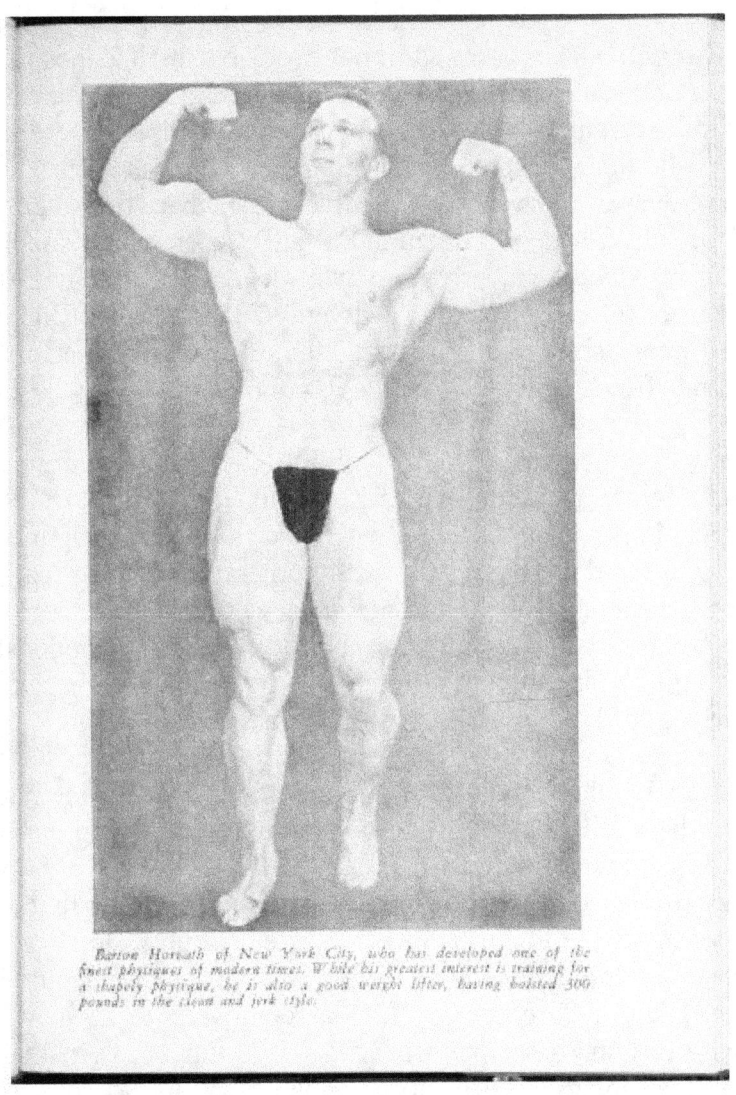

Barton Horvath of New York City, who has developed one of the finest physiques of modern times. While his greatest interest is training for a shapely physique, he is also a good weight lifter, having hoisted 300 pounds in the clean and jerk style.

Small bones, with the small knobs we have discussed, close-together bones, have prevented the Gallagher forearm from being quite as impressive as the upper arm. While the well-developed upper arm is usually twenty per cent larger than the forearm, John Gallagher's upper arm is thirty-seven per cent larger. His hips of thirty-seven and a half inches are additional proof of small bones, and his swelling chest of forty-six and a half inches is also proof that small-boned men can acquire impressive chest and shoulder developments. Starting with an eight and three-quarter inch ankle, hardly larger than the average girl's, his calves of fifteen and a half inches, while smaller than his great arm, present a well-developed, symmetrical appearance, and his thighs of twenty-four and a half inches are impressive and powerful too. He easily performs twenty-five leg presses I with 450 pounds.

Tony Terlazzo has a wrist of slightly less than seven inches and a forearm straight of 12.75. His upper arm is 15.75 (No. 2 position), which comes very, very close to the figures I have offered as the ideal measurements and the greatest expectation a man should have in developing his arm from a known wrist size. And Tony's arms are truly wonderful, the ultimate in strength and development. Johnny Terpak is fairly light boned, as evidenced by a seven-inch wrist. He has most unusual muscular power, quality of muscle as proven by the great lifts he has made; he does not have muscles of the maximum of development one would expect for his bony framework, but he does have a most exceptional development, possessing some muscles that are not seen in the forearms of other lifters I know, and a very thick development of the triceps quite close to the shoulder muscles. His forearm is 12.25 as compared to his seven-inch wrist and his upper arm 15.5—1.70 times his wrist size and the upper arm twenty-four per cent larger than his forearm. Steve Stanko's wrist is somewhat smaller than Grimek's, his forearm also a trifle smaller—14.1— but his upper arm of 16.1 is the same as Grimek's when held straight, a bit larger when flexed, but in the position we know as the No. 3, elbow held at the side. Steve and Grimek both have the same size arms—18.25; therefore Steve has nearly the ideal

82

of difference between wrist and forearm—1.85. Steve's upper arm is 22.5 per cent better than his forearm.

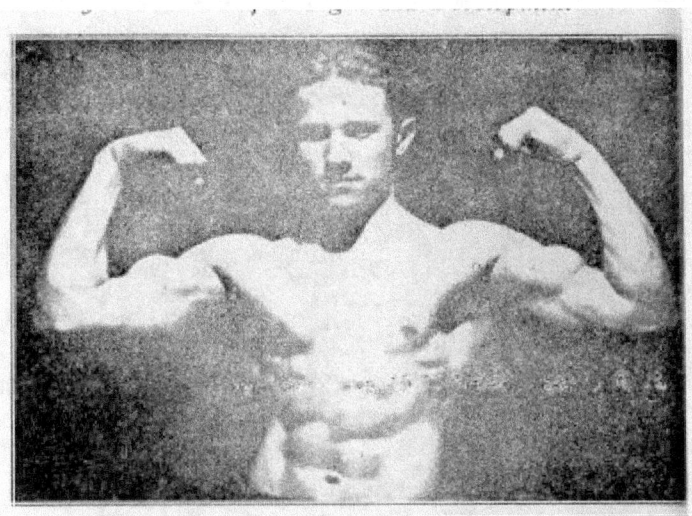

Louis Abele at 16 years of age, weight 160 pounds. When this photo was taken he had just made a lifting total of 645 pounds and we prophesied that he was a coming world's champion.

The average man who works hard—farming, logging, pick and shovel, or laboring—will have forearms which are large in comparison to the upper arms. The forearms are used constantly in performing the multitude of tasks a hard-working man must subject them to, while the upper arm seldom is operated from extreme of contraction to extreme of extension as is done in the body culturist's training. But these untrained men are not proof that my figures are not correct. I have checked them with too many figures we have on file, both of the old timers and the men who have trained but a moderate length of time. I know that you will find them to be substantially correct and if you take your own wrist size and multiply it by 1.9, you will have the forearm that is possible for you to achieve with proper training methods and if you add twenty per cent to this you will know pretty accurately the upper arm you can expect

83

to obtain. And the more strength and muscle you develop the better will be the proportion of upper arm in comparison to wrist and forearm that you will ultimately attain.

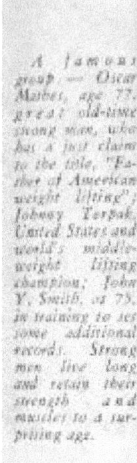

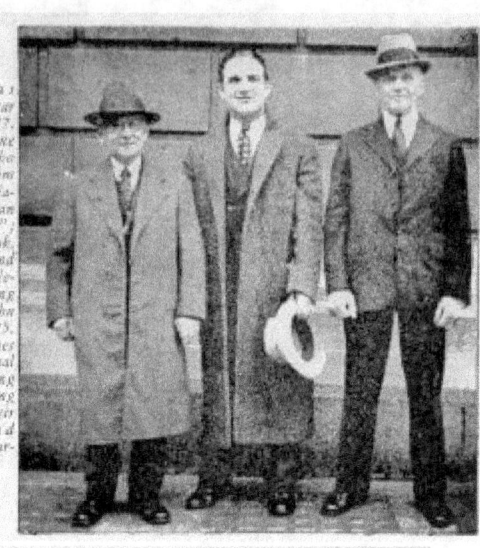

A famous group — Oscar Mathes, age 77, great old-time strong man, who has a just claim to the title, "Father of American weight lifting"; Johnny Terpak, United States and world's middleweight lifting champion; John Y. Smith, at 73, in training to set some additional records. Strong men live long and retain their strength and muscles to a surprising age.

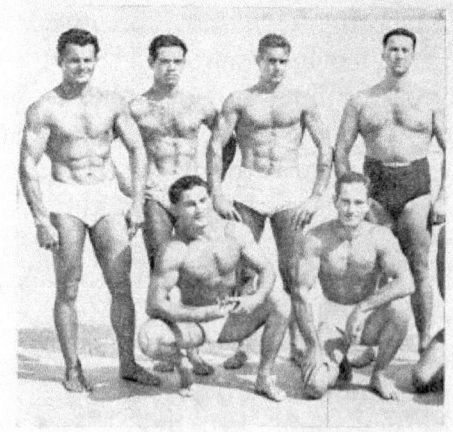

Gymnastic team of San Quentin Prison. These huskies specialize in tumbling, balancing, and weight lifting. Making good use of the York Olympic type weight-lifting set the author donated to the prison, they have built splendid physiques and superhealth in spite of their incarceration within cold walls.

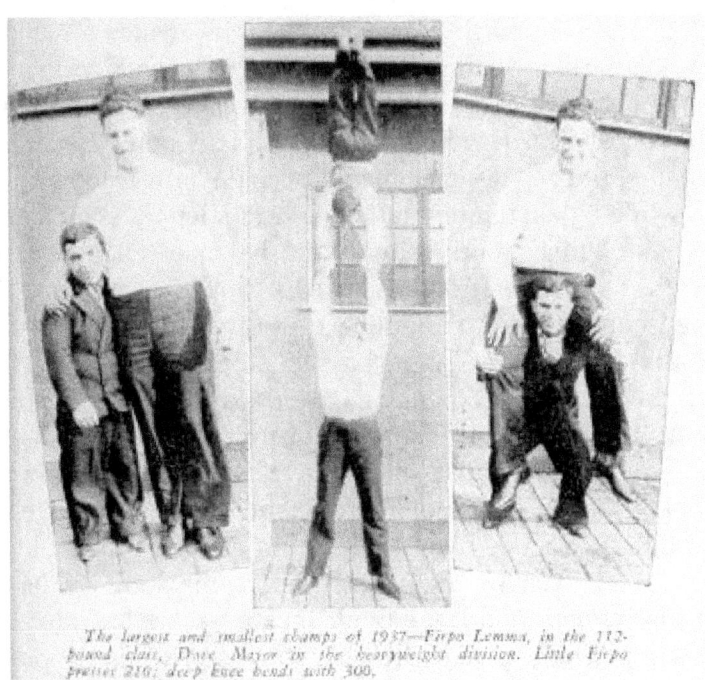

The largest and smallest champs of 1937—Firpo Lemma, in the 112-pound class, Dave Mayor in the heavyweight division. Little Firpo presses 210; deep knee bends with 300.

In considering small bones we must also give a bit of thought to short stature. We have some wonderful small men on the York team, and there have been many amazing physical specimens in the past who were short. Two of the most famous of our small lifters are Art Levan and Dick Bachtell. Art was national 126 pound champion ten consecutive years. He now weighs 140 pounds in good condition. Dick Bachtell, as mentioned before, was national 132 pound champion nine times. Dick's normal weight is 136 pounds and he has at times weighed slightly more. Both of these men are tremendously strong and good all-around athletes. How strong, is difficult for people to realize; both of these young men have put double their body weight overhead. Art performs a feat known as the Merry-Go-Round, a man sitting on his shoulders, a bar across his back, two men suspended from that, a total weight of 500 pounds, and swings them round and round. He performs a wrestler's bridge while supporting the same weight, makes a teeth lift with the largest man he can find—Gregory George, 260 pounds body weight at the last contest, does a get up with a man a great deal larger than himself. This consists of lying upon the floor pulling a man to single arm's length, and then while balancing him at single arm's length stands erect. This takes great bodily power and balance. Dick does not specialize in these strong man feats, but he is a great lifter having come within one pound of the world's record in the left arm snatch years ago, having cleaned and jerked the great weight of 273½ pounds, well over double his body weight, and is particularly adept at tumbling and balancing. Both of these young men have developed herculean proportions. The photo of Dick Bachtell which appeared on the January, 1936, cover of Strength and Health could not be excelled even by the great Grimek himself. He has an arm of fourteen and one-eighth inches— Art has an upper arm slightly larger—but Dick has the best calf development. Art is forty-one inches in chest measurement, Dick forty.

Dick and Art are five feet two in height. The average height for American men is five feet eight, so you can see that Dick and Art were meant to be little fellows. Even Tony Terlazzo is five feet four, Terpak and Elmer Farnham five feet six. None of these men permitted themselves to remain small men but have developed themselves to the point where they are miniature giants. A man of five feet four who is powerfully and symmetrically developed as is Tony Terlazzo, with sixteen-inch arms and a forty-four- inch chest, illustrates what can be done in the way of development even when the physique is average to begin with. Dick and Art equal measurements that I have come to believe are possible for most any man. I don't believe a man can be really strong unless he develops a fourteen-inch arm and a forty-inch chest. Pierre Gasnier is one great old timer who was phenomenally strong. Hardly more than five feet tall, he had a barrel-like chest and made some lifts that many larger and heavier men were unable to perform. Oscar Mathes is another of the older school of strong men who became famous in spite of a height of only four feet eleven. He was a famous strong man in 1884, even more famous a decade later and a score of years later. I receive occasional letters from him and I never cease to marvel at his beautiful handwriting. One would expect a man of seventy-six to write less perfectly than does this great little fellow. He has round red cheeks, and a biceps and other muscles which feel like iron. He is coach and counsellor of a group of young strength seekers in his own town, Lawrence, Mass. When he received a York bar bell set some time ago he reported that he just sat there for hours admiring its gleaming beauty, its perfect balance, its symmetrical design, its new and original features, and wishing that such equipment had been in existence when he was in his prime. He was puny as a child, and one of the first to prove that systematic, progressive exercise will build strength, muscle and superhealth. When in training his best weight was 105 pounds, but he did obtain some splendid measurements and perform some outstanding feats of strength. His measurements were as follows: Forearm twelve inches, with a wrist of six and a quarter inches, biceps fourteen and a half inches, chest forty inches, waist twenty-eight inches, hips thirty-five inches, thigh twenty-one inches, neck fourteen inches and calf fourteen and three-quarter inches—splendid measurements and an encouraging example for any man.

Mr. Mathes is still beautifully built, and during his professional career he was even more magnificently constructed—a miniature Hercules. Consider his proportions and how he must have looked with a forty-inch chest, a twenty-eight-inch waist, and a fourteen-and-a-half inch arm. Marvelous measurements to attain with a wrist circumference of only six and a quarter inches. This should encourage any other man to go out and do likewise, even though he feels that he is handicapped in the beginning with small bones. These measurements are very close to the ideal dimensions I have offered, his forearm in proportion to wrist being most extraordinary, more than 1.9 times his wrist, and his upper arm being twenty per cent larger than even this marvelous forearm. When you consider that most young men of average height—five feet eight—have chests of only thirty-five inches and upper arms of twelve inches, you can even better appreciate just how striking was the development of this tiny Hercules.

The majority of men who have such measurements would weigh from 150 to 160 pounds. Our weight lifting champions and near champions are exceptionally well developed, so Terpak, Terlazzo, Harrison, Farnham, and other men of this weight would have greater measurements, but most well-built and strong bar bell men would be much taller to equal the Mathes measurements.

Tony Terlazzo with his approximately sixteen-inch upper arms, depending upon the position in which he displays them, and his chest size of forty-four inches, has measurements which equal those of many larger men. His arm is only a half inch less than that of John Davis when he is lifting in the 181 pound class. The smaller men too, while not lifting quite as much as the bigger fellows, do closely approach their records. The small bent pressers are not too far back of the larger men. Val De Genaro with a press of 215 in the 148 pound class compared to the nation's best bent presser, Bob Harley, who, weighing 180 pounds, pressed 254; Terlazzo's world record press of 255 compared with Stanko's best press of 290; Terlazzo's clean and jerk of 340 compared to Stanko's 375—all additional proof that the small, light-boned man need not despair. He can build himself into a powerhouse with measurements and strength records which closely approach those of the big fellows. A good big man is better than a good little man, but a trained little man is better than an untrained or partially trained big man.

Back to Oscar Mathes again. He performed some feats of strength which seem unbelievable. It is reported that he made a standing broad jump record of ten feet seven inches. Really incredible. The best jumpers of the York Bar Bell Club are sensational enough, with Terpak, Harrison, Davis and Grimek jumping ten feet or more; Grimek without training propelling his huge body through ten feet six inches of space. Dick Bachtell, little taller than Mathes, and a great all-around performer, has jumped eight feet five inches. Broad jumping is a real test of strength. The vital portion of the body, the lower back, the development of which is the result of weight lifting exercises, also provides the muscles which propel the body forward in broad jumping. All strong men are good jumpers and good runners too.

Small-boned men may find it difficult to build the forearms and the calves, two of the more difficult portions of the body to develop, but they have no difficulty in building broader shoulders, bigger chests, large thighs and upper arms. The calf of the leg is the despair of many body build-ers. They obtain splendid and satisfactory proportions in other parts of their bodies but their calves insist on lagging in development. This is controlled in great measure by the bone size and the construction of the ankle. Some men have more favorable foot and ankle leverage than others and thus do not need and cannot develop calf muscles of satisfactory size. This is proven by observing the calves of sprinters and high jumpers. In recent years many of the best performers in these sports have been negroes. Originally the negroes came from various parts of Africa. The Masai in northern

Kenya Colony are tall, most males being over six feet in height. Some are nearly seven. They are great jumpers: it is reported that a number of them could break the world's record in the high jump with a leap of at least seven feet. In their own intertribal competitions they leap from a raised platform, and hop over the bar at a height of approximately eight feet. But they do not obtain worthy calf development in spite of their great running and jumping ability. In the south of this large colony and in most of central and tropical Africa, there are tribes such as the Akikuyu who are shorter, heavier, darker, who have well-developed calves. The first tribesmen and their descendants can train to the point of being world's champions in jumping and sprinting and have little calf development, while the latter tribesmen with little or no effort will have unusual development of the calves. In the same manner the South Sea Islanders have marvelous pectoral or chest muscle development with little effort on their part. These are inherited traits and it is difficult to completely overcome such an inherited physical characteristic. But once again I repeat that practically none of us are of such pure stock that we have these definite inherited characteristics. If your lower leg bone is quite long, there is less chance of obtaining a satisfactory calf development than if it is shorter and stockier. Everything has its compensations however. If you have long leg bones you'll become strong, have unusual power, speed and explosive energy in these muscles. As a result of training you will obtain your fair share of physical benefit.

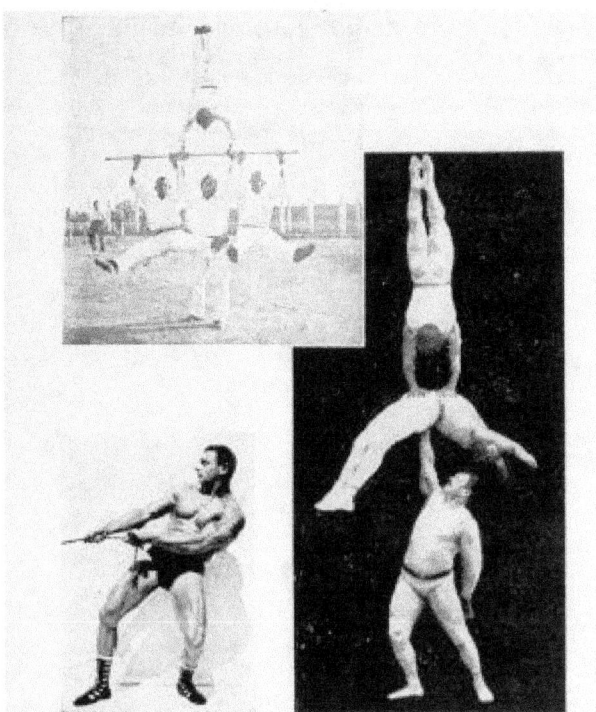

A powerful European strong man holding over 500 pounds aloft. It is proof of strength and balancing skill to hold one man overhead with one hand, but add to this another man in the hand stand position and the feat is truly stupendous. The small photo is of Siegmund Klein, famous American bar bell instructor who conducts one of the finest gyms in the world, in New York City.

Regardless of your height, the size of your wrists and ankles, your hips—all evidence of the size of your bones— you can accomplish what you desire in a physical way. Ambition, proper application to the right progressive training methods and persistence will bring you physical improvements of which you can be justly proud. Where would Mr. Mathes have been if he had despaired because he was so much smaller than most girls? But he persisted until he performed strength feats of the most amazing magnitude. At one time he lifted with the hands alone a barrel weighing 513 pounds, carried it from a platform eighteen inches high and moved it ten feet to another which was twenty-four inches in height—a great height for a man of his short stature.

CHAPTER FIVE
Tendon and Ligament Strength

A CHAIN is no stronger than its weakest link, and this brings up a discussion of the basis of true power, the strength of the tendons and particularly the ligaments. A great many people believe that muscular size is all that matters in considering the strength of a man, that if he has large measurements he must be correspondingly strong. This is not necessarily true, for the determining factor is just how have the muscles been developed? If the sizeable measurements have resulted from high repetitions with tension methods, inflated tissue, which is never as strong as real muscle made with heavy methods, prob ably accounts for the measurement. Such muscles which look good to the unpracticed eye are the result of high repetitions and constant flexing or tension. While such exercises swell the tissue and make larger measurements, the resulting muscle consists of a coarser structure which is never particularly strong.

In the chapter, "Quality of Muscle," you will obtain good reasons concerning the unusual strength of some men as compared to others with similar measurements and apparently identical muscular development. But there is a great difference, as is observed constantly in comparing two pieces of steel or comparing iron and steel. The piece of steel which has been treated under heat in a variety of ways is so much stronger than an even more bulky piece of iron. Iron is coarser than steel, yet not so strong; similarly the coarser tissues of the inflated muscle do not permit it to contract as forcefully as the better made muscle with superior quality, and without this powerful contraction it is not so strong.

93

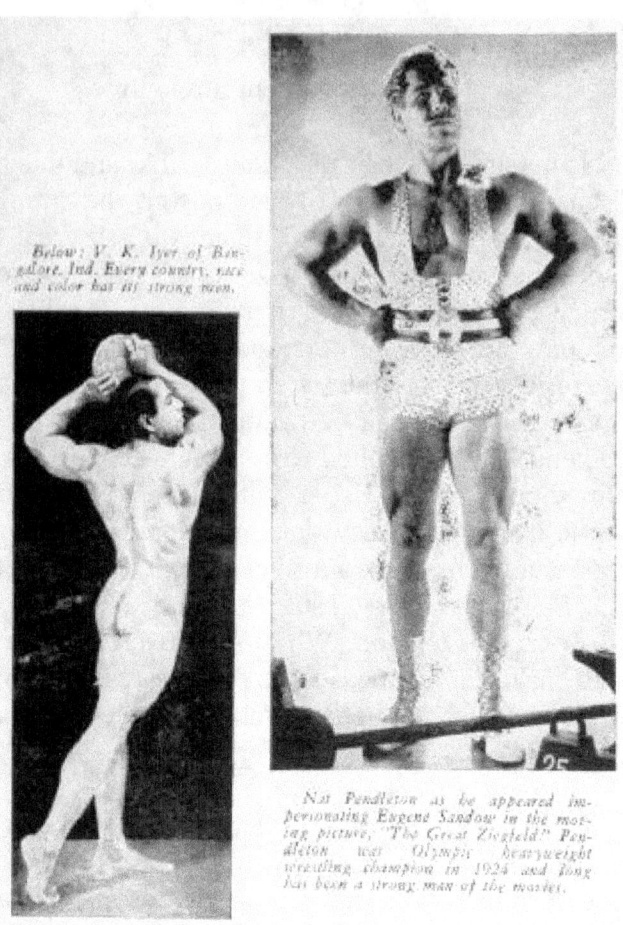

Below: V. K. Iyer of Bangalore, Ind. Every country, race and color has its strong men.

Nat Pendleton as he appeared impersonating Eugene Sandow in the moving picture, "The Great Ziegfeld." Pendleton was Olympic heavyweight wrestling champion in 1924 and long has been a strong man of the movies.

But that is only one reason why the man who has pumped up his muscles with light tensing movements is not as strong as the man who has acquired his strength through heavier methods. With inflated tissue there has been no real stress applied to the muscles at any time. The attachments of these muscles—the tendons—have not become strong and tough and are unable to grasp the bone to which they are attached with sufficient force to withstand a heavy stress placed upon them when there is an attempt to make a heavy lift. Incredible as it may seem, I have seen many of these men who had developed what they and some of their friends considered to be a nice physique with light methods, who actually could not hang with one hand from a chinning bar. Similarly they could not pick up a heavy dumbell or a bar bell with one hand, a weight which would not be burdensome for the man with all-around development. In spite of the increased size of muscles which have been obtained by tensing methods these men are not a bit stronger than the attachments of the muscles which connect with the ligaments and the tendons.

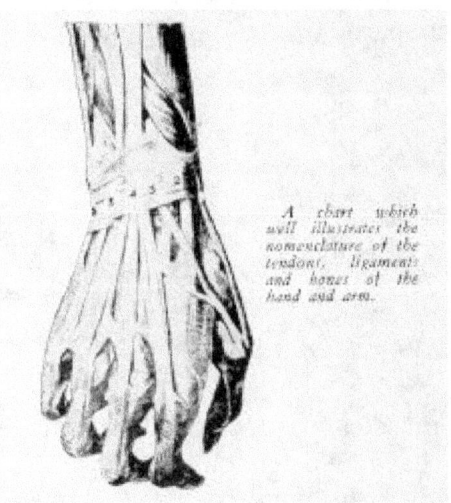

A chart which well illustrates the nomenclature of the tendons, ligaments and bones of the hand and arm.

The men who use faulty training methods do not have balanced strength or development and fail when their muscles are put to the test.

I have had so many letters from men of this type. They have exercised for long months with their constant extension and compression of the muscles, until some day they come in contact with a bar bell and then are much surprised to find that their friend who does manual work, but is lighter than they and apparently not as well developed, is able to lift 400 pounds in the dead weight lift while they can't handle 300; their friend lifts 150 pounds overhead while ninety pounds is the limit of their strength. And then the trained man who owns the bar bell quickly demonstrates that he can lift 550 pounds in the dead weight style and put 250 pounds overhead in the method commonly known as the two hands clean and jerk. The man with the inflated tissue likes to feel that he lacks knack, but what he really lacks is strength in the attachments, the tendons and ligaments. Let's study for a few moments the work that these ligaments and attachments are designed to do, before we continue with proper exercises for strengthening these all-important parts.

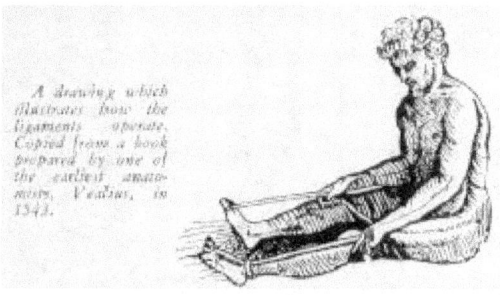

A drawing which illustrates how the ligaments operate. Copied from a book prepared by one of the earliest anatomists, Vesalius, in 1543.

Nearly all muscles, particularly those which are fastened to the bones, have two tendons at the ends. These serve as hands to grasp the bone so that the muscle can exert its force, thus moving the bone and the body in the manner desired. The tendon never contracts, it just transmits the pull. Many body builders believe, when it does not increase in size as do the muscles, that it is not necessary to exercise in such a manner that the tendons will be strengthened. Muscles are made to use, not to look at, and there should be a full share of exercises included in any training program to strengthen the tendons and the ligaments.

Like the variance in the length of muscles there is considerable variation in the length of tendons. Some are very short, others are more than twelve inches long, as for example the tendons of the fingers which make it possible for me to rattle this typewriter so merrily this morning. These long tendons may be seen by closely examining the muscle chart. In one of these muscles the body, or as it is often called the belly of the muscle, is eight inches long and located in the forearm; the tendons are merely two inches long at the upper or proximal end. Thousands of white fibres of connective tissue, all parallel and arranged in bundles, constitute the body of such a tendon. Among the white fibres are a few elastic fibres; attached to these for their upkeep and repair are constructive cells or fibroblasts which have played a part in their formation. A bluish iridescence is characteristic of the tendons. Each of these tiny tendon fibres is attached at one end to a muscle fibre. The joint is so tightly cemented that all the force of the muscle can never break away from its tendinous end. In the case of torn muscles, of which you have sometimes heard, the muscle fibre will tear in two, but never will there be a separation from the tendon or from the attachment of the tendon. From this brief description it must be evident that the real strength of the body lies in the tendons and their partners or counterparts, the ligaments. The injury, always a painful one, is called, in athletic parlance, a pulled muscle or a "Charley horse."

A delicate sheath of connective tissue surrounds the tendon in which the blood for nourishment, lymphatic vessels for carrying off the debris, injured, dead, worn out cells, tissues and nerves, are contained. While there are some muscle fibres in the belly of a large muscle which never reach a tendon, every fibre of the tendon is fastened to some muscle fibre. The pull of the muscles which are not fastened to a tendon is made through the connective tissue sheath which transmits the power of the muscle. These connective tissue sheaths which are a necessary part of the muscular construction are made of white fibres and elastic fibres. Excessive expansion of the muscles is prevented by these white fibres which run crosswise around the belly of the muscle. A muscle contracts in the middle in proportion to its contraction in length, it must be remembered. The white fibres also run lengthwise at the ends of the muscle aiding in the transmission of the pull to the tendon. The work of the elastic fibres is to aid the fibres in attaining a position of rest and relaxation after the contraction is completed.

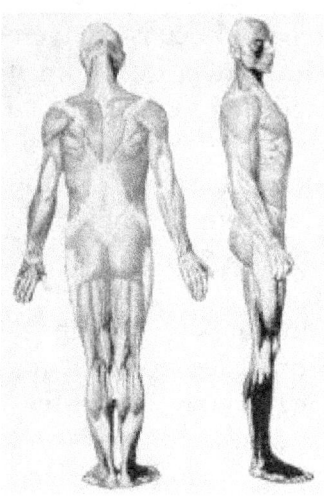

Beauty and perfection in the mechanical adjustment are revealed when a study is made of the length and position of the tendons and the size and position of the body of the muscles. Where it is necessary to overlay one muscle with another which is done so often, particularly in the complex arrangement of the muscles of the limbs, but also in muscles of the sides which must be prepared to hold the body erect, bend powerfully from side to side, or move with a twisting action, some of the muscles are most likely to be tendinous. The reason for this is the fact that there is not room for a muscle to contract in a normal manner without interfering with the action of other and perhaps more important muscles. An example of this condition would be where the breast muscles cover the upper and tendinous end of the biceps. The muscles are invariably tendinous opposite the joints where thick masses of muscle fibre would interfere with bending and twisting. Some muscles are classed as omohyoid because they extend in two directions and must exert their pull in these diverse manners. Such a muscle is found at the side of the neck, and the Sartorius muscle of the leg, a muscle which runs round the other muscles from a position on the inner and lower thigh to the front and top of the other side of the thigh. This muscle, often called the "Tailor muscle," is flat in construction while the muscle first mentioned is tendinous in the center to facilitate its action.

The masses of the muscles are disposed around the bones in such a manner that when properly developed they not only produce limbs of beauty and shapeliness but are practical in shape and size. Frequently I write that a development commensurate with the size of the bones and the proportions of the skeletal framework will be obtained. No man ever had too much muscle. John Grimek has, as all body builders know, a most herculean development. Yet these huge muscles are so beautifully designed that the Grimek physique is most pleasing to the eye, and so practically arranged that he can perform feats of actual contortion, such as standing on a box and touching the floor with his hands, knees held stiff, fifteen inches lower than his feet, touching his elbows while holding the legs stiff, performing a full split, and demonstrating many twisting and turning movements which illustrate his supreme flexibility, efficiency of muscle, and at the same time prove that a trained man cannot obtain too much muscle, sufficient muscle which could hinder him in work or athletics as some pseudo experts would have us believe.

These men who are slow and called "muscle bound" are invariably men who are untrained, only partially trained or have acquired such a development through moving their muscles over only a slight range as is done in many phases of work. But the seeker of strength and development who follows my training methods will in every exercise operate his muscles over their complete range, from extreme contraction to extreme extension, and thus retain flexibility and maximum length in spite of their size.

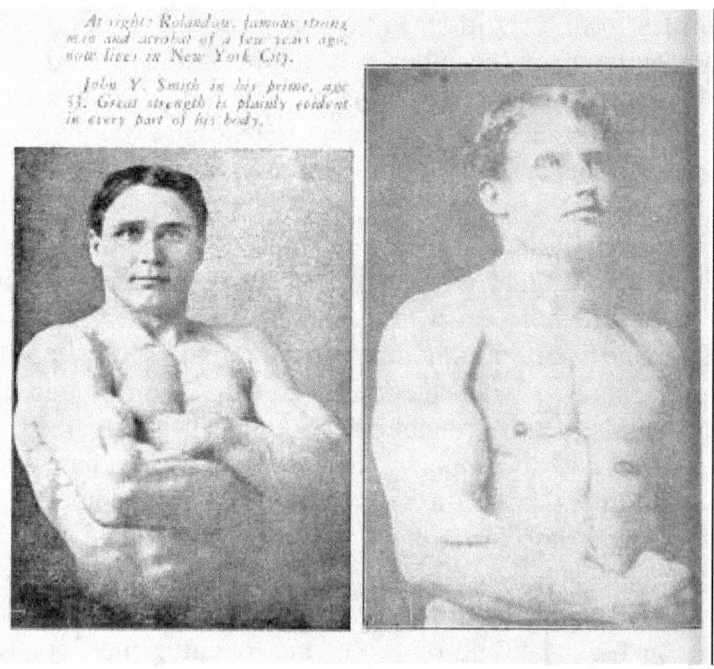

At right: Roland *an, famous strong man and acrobat of a few years ago, now lives in New York City.

John Y. Smith in his prime, age 33. Great strength is plainly evident in every part of his body.

If you study anatomy just a bit, you will be impressed, really thrilled, at the splendid work nature has done in designing the muscle nomenclature of the various animals which inhabit this world. The amazing muscular ability of all representatives of the cat family—the tiger, lion, jaguar, leopard, puma and even our miniature feline, but a smaller model nevertheless of the big cats, the domestic Tommy or

Tabby Cat—is astonishing to contemplate. They have strength, speed, power, smooth, silent, muscular action, can jump many times their length, and a cat dropped from the top of the Washington Monument landed without a broken bone. They possess strength, balance and flexibility to the nth degree. Or consider the difference in construction of the beautiful, fiery, prancing stallion. Isn't it a marvel of muscular beauty? With these and so many other animals which could be mentioned the muscles are admirably suited and adapted mechanically to perform their functions.

When necessary, muscle masses must be placed far from the parts they are designed to control; then they are connected by long tendons. In such cases the ligaments come into use. Where these long tendons pass over a joint, to prevent them from pulling away from their proper position, or from sliding sideways in bending movements, the tendons are held down by ligaments which are placed opposite the joints. The tendons also slide through grooves in the bone, but the ligaments must be responsible for the maintenance of their proper position. This is particularly difficult in the case of muscles which operate over two or more joints. Like the muscles of the fingers, which in many cases are in the forearm, there are long tendons which actually operate over six joints. Many heavy ligaments hold these tendons in position as you can see in the anatomical charts. Very few men have ever had the development of the tendons and ligaments that the great old timer, John Y. Smith, possesses. Hold out your hand, bend the fingers up so that you can see the tendons; while the ligaments are not seen they are there just the same holding the tendons to the joints. When you look at the palms of your hands, the chances are a thousand to one that you see only the lines of the skin and the muscles. But if you had the opportunity to see the palms of the hands of the Boston Strong Man, almost an octogenarian, you would see tendons just as prominently displayed on the inside of his hands. One would believe that he had two sets of tendons, one set for the front of the hand, the other for the back, but it is only the superdevelopment of these tendons, the result of much heavy training, training which has proven that tendons and ligaments are the basis of true strength, and has brought much honor to Smith.

Old time strong men would supplement the strength of their wrists by wearing wrist straps. While these formed a protection, they had a tendency actually to weaken the wrist and it is better not to use leather wrist straps. The ligaments of the wrist wrap around the tendons in a manner similar to the effect of a wrist strap. Our champion lifters, handling as they do from 300 to Steve Stanko's 375 world record poundage, hold this great weight at the shoulders with the hands turned back and all the strain on the ligaments. Then with a great heave of the legs, shoulders and arms the weight is jerked to arm's length overhead. It is evident that the ligaments of the wrists must be tremendously powerful. It is possible, and is done frequently by European lifters in particular, to add additional support to these ligaments by wrapping bandage cloth around the wrist. It should be applied loosely enough so that it is not tight when the wrists are straight, but will offer some support when the wrist is bent back sustaining the great weight that modern lifters handle. The best men of our team, who hold the national and world's records, do not find it necessary to have such support; their training has brought the tendons and ligaments to such an advanced state of strength that they per. form their work without apparent effort.

In the wrists and ankles the ligaments have the most complex work to perform. They are connected in such a manner that they form a continuous ligamentous tunnel on the palmar side of the hand through which the tendons glide. Copied from the earliest known, partially authentic book on anatomy, is shown a simple, crude, but nevertheless realistic drawing, illustrating how the ligaments operate. This illustration was published nearly four centuries ago in a book by Vealius, prepared in 1543.

Muscular size means little without accompanying strength in ligaments and tendons. There is a relationship between the three—muscles, ligaments and tendons. Its ability to contract under great pressure and to exert great force is the chief value of the muscle. This powerful action would be useless if it were not applied to the bones by equal strength in tendons and ligaments. With strength in this triumvirate of muscle, tendons and ligaments, a weight lifter, other athlete or working man can be successful in a heavy test of strength. All muscular contraction is performed by the vigorous pulling of the muscles, the sinewy levers, the tendons and restraining force of the ligaments. As each group of muscles operate, exert their force through shortening, the ligaments operate or lever, and unless they are strong enough to help the muscles do the work required of them, great contractile power of the muscles and success in the work desired whether it be climbing a rope, chinning a bar or lifting a weight is not possible.

The final test of strength is the united effort of the muscles and the tendons and ligaments. A good comparison for the similarity between ligament and muscular strength and the manner in which they must operate together can be seen in watching a derrick or crane in action. In this case the power is provided by the motor; it applies its power through the derrick boom, and the cable which imparts this power is similar to the tendons and ligaments. No matter how powerful the motor may be, if the strength of the derrick boom and the cables was not equal to it, only a fraction of

103

the load of which the motor is capable could be lifted. And in the body you can lift no more than your ligaments will withstand. They should always have a surplus of power, able to perform much more than the effort which the muscles can put forth. This balance of power which is necessary in the derrick, and also in the muscles and attachments, illustrates the folly of body culturists who spend all their time devdoping the muscles in such a manner that the ligaments and tendons receive little strengthening effect.

You can test your ligament strength in two ways. The best known would be to perform a dead weight lift with the knuckles front. Here the weight lifted depends entirely on the gripping power, which of course is controlled by the strength of the ligaments and tendons. While the record in this style is only 550, when the bar is held with the palms facing each other, John Terry has hoisted 600 pounds; the world's heavyweight record is 657, held by Carl Pepke. One of the best dead weight lifting records made by a modern strength star was established by Walter Podolak— 652 pounds—who is now a professional wrestler. Podolak is a short, broad, big-chested powerhouse who would have gone far as a weight lifter had he not become a professional wrestler.

Another way to test the power of ligaments and tendons is to jerk a weight somewhat near your limit to arm's length overhead, then lower the weight slowly. At various stages of the lowering of the bell stop for a few seconds and see how long you can hold it. If you are the possessor of very strong tendons more than likely you can hold the weight of the bell, but if it comes down slowly at first and then with a rush, you will know that you are lacking in attachment strength.

A few experts believed at one time that the failure of some lifters to hold a weight overhead was solely the result of weak tendons and ligaments. But the real difficulty is the fact that some individuals are so constructed that their bones are not in direct line, or actually bent in in a knock- kneed manner. Luhaar, the great Esthonian lifter who held the world's clean and jerk record for some years at 369 pounds—before big Steve Stanko elevated it still farther to its point as this is written at 375—had arms which bent in more than the arms of any of the world's leading lifters whom I have seen. Of the York champions who have the greatest trouble in locking their arms, Eddie Harrison, who has been runner up to world's champion Tony Terlazzo year after year in the lightweight class, and Dick Bachtell, who is the oldest man at present in point of years of service in amateur weight lifting, have lost most honors due to this unfortunate physical characteristic. A man can't have everything, but this condition is a handicap. Mike Mongiola, who won the 126-pound national title the first year that Art Levan of the York team abdicated his throne after a ten-year winning streak—the longest in the history of amateur weight lifting—has a similar difficulty. The only possible solution of this problem is to develop the power of ligaments and tendons so that the weight can be held overhead for the referee's count of two by muscular and attachment strength alone, and by holding the bar with a much wider than usual grip. This changes the position of the elbow joint, applying the pressure in a different manner and frequently makes it possible to hold the weight for the count.

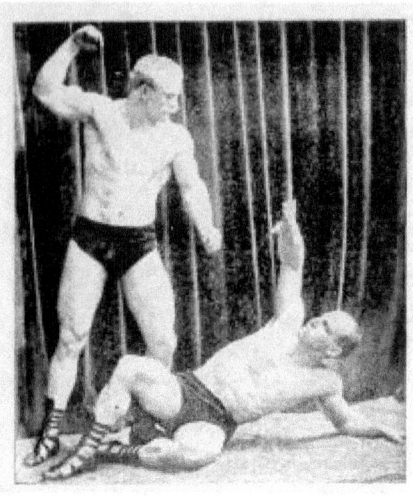

I have always been a claimant of the title, world's worst presser. I have an unfavorable condition of leverage that has been impossible to overcome. To my knowledge, I am the only man in the world history of weight lifting who has jerked to arm's length, after cleaning the weight, double what he could press. All during my lifting career I was nearly double in the clean and jerk as compared to what I could press: the first year 80 press and 150 clean and jerk when I first received my bar bell, a year later 115 press and 225 clean and jerk, more years later 135 press and 265 clean and jerk, in my first contest after a serious auto accident, 121 press and 236 clean and jerk (a near success with the next weight, 242, which I cleaned, would have given me double in the clean and jerk as compared to what I had pressed), but more years later 145 press and 295 clean and jerk—the first time I officially lifted double in the clean and jerk what I could press. Unfavorable leverage in the press which robs me of maximum pressing power, short upper arm, long lower arm, handicaps my pressing from the shoulder. In an endeavor to overcome this condition I performed special exercises to strengthen the ligaments— the Jefferson or straddle lift notably, but also holding the heavily loaded bar overhead. I rigged up an overhead pair of chains about six inches lower than the bar would be when held at arm's length. I would practice getting under the bar and holding it at arm's length; this taught the mus- cles to properly adjust themselves to balance and sustain the weight overhead. From the position with weight at arm's length I would lower it slowly, at times trying to sus- tain it after the arms had been bent. The weight could not come down more than six inches so there was no danger of dropping it upon me. I quickly developed the ability to sus- tain a great deal more weight than I could jerk overhead, finally succeeding in holding 325 pounds overhead in the strength feat known as the continental and jerk behind neck. I have been successful in pressing out most any sort of a weight if I don't get it high enough in the initial jerk to fix it at arm's length. I have pressed out 300 pounds in this manner a number of times in spite of my unfavorable press- ing leverage. All good proof that I have developed a high degree of ligament strength. I am known as the man who never misses a jerk and it is so long since I missed one that I have forgotten when.

There are men who have great sustaining power and in- variably they are the possessors of powerful muscular at- tachments. Shorter, stockier men usually can jerk a great deal of weight and easily hold it overhead. Joseph Manger, the Olympic heavyweight lifting champion, jerked 408 pounds to arm's length with comparative ease at the time he came to this country as a member of the German team who lifted against our United States team. Gregory George^ known as the St. Louis Samson, while having arms so huge that he finds difficulty in holding the bar at the chest, can jerk most any weight when once it has been lifted to his shoulders. One night he jerked 360 three times from the shoulder, this being the most weight available. I am con- fident that he could jerk 400. While weaker in the jerk than in the clean in the beginning, increased strength, the result of constant heavy training, has placed Stanko at the point where he never misses a jerk.

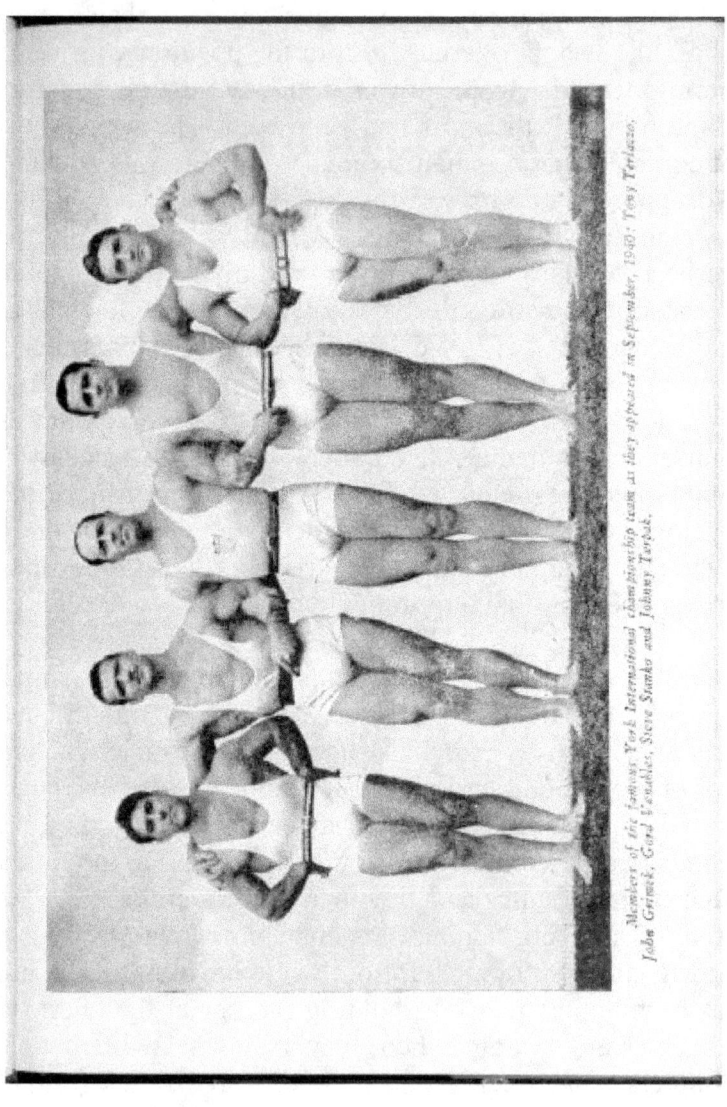

Members of the famous York International championship team as they appeared in September, 1940 : Tony Terlazzo, John Grimek, Gord Venables, Steve Stanko and Johnny Terpak.

Another who does not have good jerking form but possesses the ability to elevate great weights overhead is John Grimek. He has jerked 375 to arm's length, and his jerk is a heave and a press out. Grimek has the most amazing development of the attachments of the wrist, and the ankle too, but we are discussing chiefly the muscles used in overhead lifting. Grimek has a wrist so huge and developed that people who see it wonder at first if it has not been broken or injured in some way. But it is this size due to unusual strength in first the tendons and then the ligaments. Grimek, to maintain his present strength and physique, trains less than any man I know. When he does train he uses extremely heavy poundages, weights that are surprising. In the side bend exercise I have seen him take the famous Cyr Bell, which is one of the special fixtures in our gymnasium, and perform ten bends with it loaded to 248½ pounds. Many men use fifteen pounds or perhaps twenty- five if they feel particularly strong in this movement, so it's evident that they cannot hope to equal the strength and development of a man like Grimek unless they constantly advance to the point of handling more and more weight.

When a man has trained himself by strength methods you can see this without putting him to the test by examining chiefly his wrists, which are the most visible; for thick ligaments, the mark of a really strong man, display themselves around the joints.

All men who have really well-developed forearms have a very thick arm right up to the wrist, the result of tendon development. When ligaments are weak the joints are weak I too, for the ligaments, while holding the muscle in its proper position at the joints, also strengthen the joint. What the muscles gain by increased contraction the ligaments must also gain by increased power of leverage. Exercises which employ the ligaments to their fullest capacity will develop thicker and of course stronger ligaments. The exercises need not be many, nor be continued over many repetitions, but heavy weights must be sustained, exercises which require the maximum of strength of the ligaments and attachments. The practice of such exercises without muscle building movements will build powerful but stringy arms which are not so strong looking except to the student of strength and anatomy who knows where to look for the strength of a man.

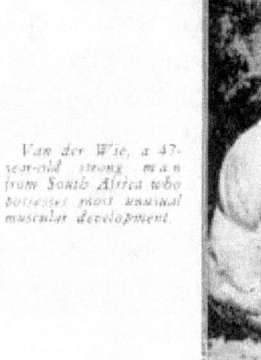

Van der Wie, a 47-year-old strong man from South Africa who possesses most unusual muscular development.

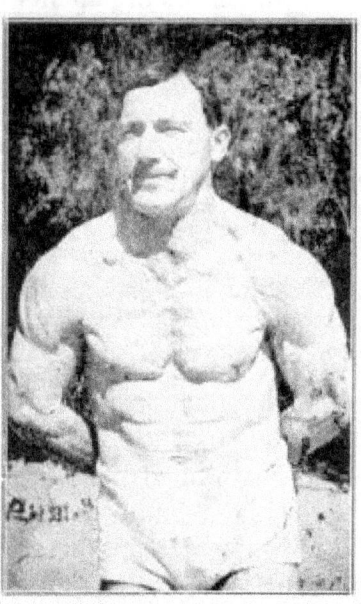

Among the old timers who had unusual ligament strength were Herman Gorner, the great South African German professional strong man, Saxon, Maxick, Steinborn, Aston, and Hackenschmidt, and of course today any one of the weight lifting champions or near champions would be a fine example of this important form of strength. Among the old timers it was evident that Warren Lincoln Travis ranked well at the head of the list for I saw him perform a two finger lift, a world's record, with 830 pounds, a tremendous

110

poundage, which could be sustained only with the greatest of tendon and ligament strength. Such a weight would tear the muscles and attachments of a man less strong.

From the discussion contained in this chapter it is evident that you should at times in your training handle very heavy poundages, not only for muscle building, but for developing the strength of tendons and ligaments—exercises such as the one and two hands dead lifts, the straddle lift, and sustaining weights overhead.

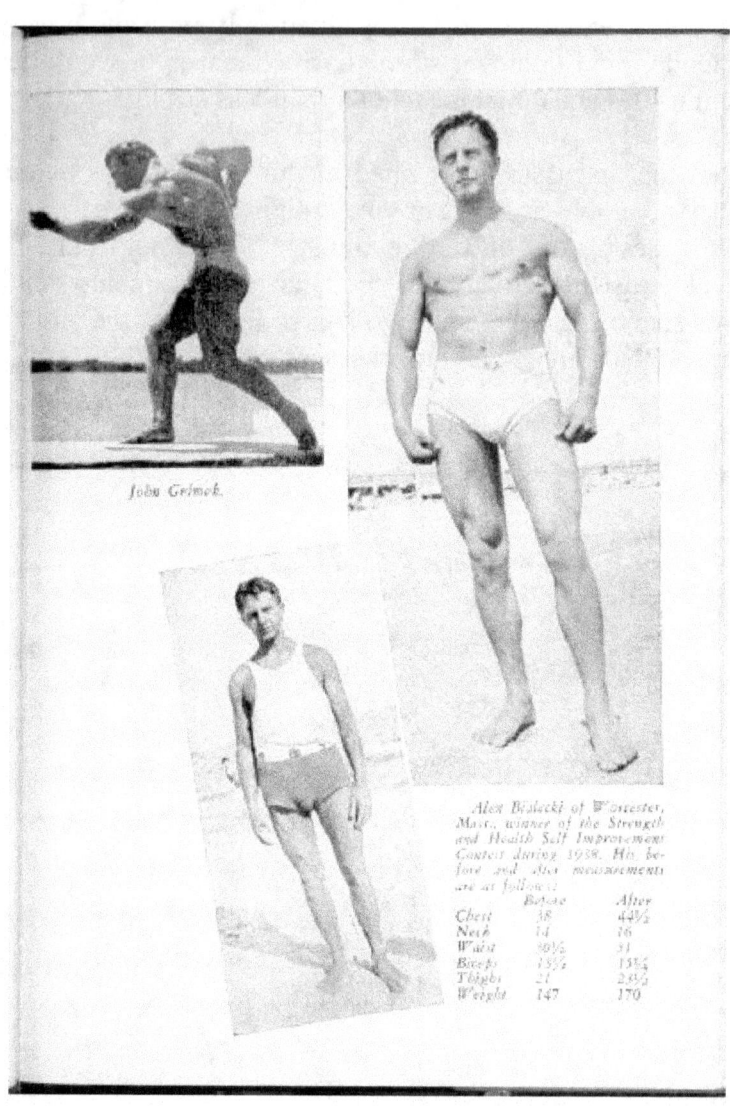

John Grimek.

Alex Bialecki of Worcester,
Mass., winner of the Strength
and Health Self Improvement
Contest during 1938. His before and after measurements
are as follows:

	Before	After
Chest	38	44½
Neck	14	16
Waist	30½	31
Biceps	13½	15¾
Thighs	21	23½
Weight	147	170

CHAPTER SIX
Importance of Size and Weight

A good big man is always better than a good little man, but, as I wrote elsewhere in this book, a trained and skilled little man is better than an undeveloped big man. This is particularly evident in strength sports such as weight lifting, for the smaller champions can lift more than any except the very best of the bigger lifters. The average fairly strong man, if put to the test, can press 100 pounds; most young fellows who think they are fairly strong can put up about 120 pounds. Bigger men who have built muscles through hard work can occasionally hoist 150 pounds. Some years ago the York Bar Bell Company had a display of weights and other equipment at the local county fair. Sometimes as many as a hundred thousand people attend this fair on Thursday, the big day. To create additional interest a prize was offered to any untrained man who could put 150 pounds overhead with two hands. During the entire week some hundreds of men of all ages tried, but only two who were really untrained, as far as weight lifting was concerned, were able to lift 150 pounds or more overhead. One of these had been a professional hand balancer years before and could not be considered an untrained man when he pressed 150 pounds with some help from the legs. Another man elevated 160 pounds, but he was employed in a flour mill and it was his work to pile up the heavy bags of flour. Frequently they were placed higher than his head and his muscles had become strong enough to lift these bags overhead. He made the best record of the entire week's demonstration with a lift of 160 pounds. But even he could not be considered an untrained man, for he has been lifting not iron weights, 'tis true, but weight in another form— flour.

In my entire experience with weight lifting, at present ranging over a period of eighteen years, I have seen several men make creditable lifts the first try. Most untrained men can pull a fair weight to the shoulders, but few of them have any pressing or jerking ability. Coming back from the Olympic Games one of the colored boxers, a 170-pound man, pulled 209 to the chest, but he was unable to get it from there overhead. This is the best lift I have witnessed on the part of a man who has not had special training.

When Tony Terlazzo steps out and presses 255 pounds, as he did to establish his astounding world's record in the 148 pound class, we see an example of the good little man who is better than the untrained or partially trained big man. Only a handful of men in this country, regardless of body weight, lift as much overhead in the two hands clean and jerk as does Tony. In fact this small but mighty lifter has made a lifting total of 830 (his best lifts would total 845), and 830 is the same aggregate total lifted by the Olympic heavyweight champion, Skobla, of Czechoslovakia, at the Los Angeles Olympics in 1932. Tony himself could only "put up" seventy pounds in the two hands lift when he started with weight lifting, so the great results he has attained and the fine build and muscular development with symmetrical proportions he has developed are solely the result of physical training.

But you couldn't expect as small a man as Tony Terlazzo to lift with the very best of the big men—fellows like the senior national champion, Steve Stanko, or last year's junior national champion and Stanko's leading competitor, Louis Abele, for these men have skill, development, and greater size and weight. The smaller men are much better in proportion to body weight than the bigger fellows, similar to the ant which is far stronger in proportion to size than is an elephant, but the trained good big man, with his added weight and power, will outlift the smaller men.

We have a similar condition in wrestling. There are some remarkable small wrestlers who can defeat ordinary wrestlers in the heavyweight class. Otto Arco, weight 140 or slightly more, made a good showing in open European competition in wrestling years ago. He could not beat the very best of the big men, but he did beat many big men. When the little fellow is very strong it's almost impossible to throw him, although he may not have the power to toss a larger wrestler. Coming back from the Olympics there were a number of members of the wrestling team who tried unsuccessfully to pin some of our 148- and 165-pound lifters, without success. The lifters were so strong that they could wiggle or writhe out of all holds. So many of the big wrestlers one sees today are little more than actors, put on a good show, but are not skilled as wrestlers or very well developed. Smaller men, weight-trained men such as Jesse James, the York Bar Bell man who won the world's light-heavyweight wrestling title, or Dr. "Drop Kick" Murphy, another great light-heavyweight who uses York weights, or Walter Stratton, also prominent as a light-heavy wrestler for these many years, who also carries a set of York weights with him in his travels, weigh about 175 pounds. These 175-pound wrestlers overcome many of the 200- to 250-pound wrestlers, but they cannot beat the best of the really big men. For many years Jim Londos has been the heavyweight wrestling king. He started by being a little fellow (he's hardly five feet six tall); through weight training and wrestling he built a wonderful 200-pound body which made it possible for him to overcome much bigger men and win the world's title. But when Jesse James, the world's best at 175, met Londos, the world's champion, outweighing him more than twenty-five pounds, after a great battle he lost to a good, bigger man.

In boxing the smallest men no matter how good they may be could not be expected to fight the really big fellows on equal terms. They strike hard blows, harder in proportion to their weight than the big fellows, but the larger men have an advantage of weight and power which they cannot overcome. Henry Armstrong, at one time the boxing king in three weight divisions, would have no chance at all against Joe Louis. Joe would find it difficult to catch up with Armstrong, but Armstrong could not hurt Louis. Yet there are a great many cases of smaller boxers meeting and defeating all comers when they travelled with the circus or a fair. A case here of a good little man beating ordinary big men.

One of the old timers who was small but extremely powerful was Joe Wolcott, the old-time colored fighter. He weighed only 145 pounds but was so strong that he was often called the Giant Killer. He beat so many of the larger fellows that it became very difficult to obtain matches for him. Harry Greb, who seldom weighed more than 160 pounds, met the best of them, including Gene Tunney, shortly before the ex-marine won the world's heavyweight title from Jack Dempsey in the rain at the Sesquicentennial in Philadelphia back in 1926. Mickey Walker, the "Toy Bulldog" of Elizabeth, N. J., world's middleweight champion, met some good heavyweights. In the beginning he was tall enough to weigh, as an average man, 140, yet he developed such power in his small body that he beat many good big men. But if he were to fight Jack Dempsey at his best, if both would start a blow at the same time, and both connected simultaneously, the greater weight and power of Dempsey would inflict the superior damage upon the chin of his opponent.

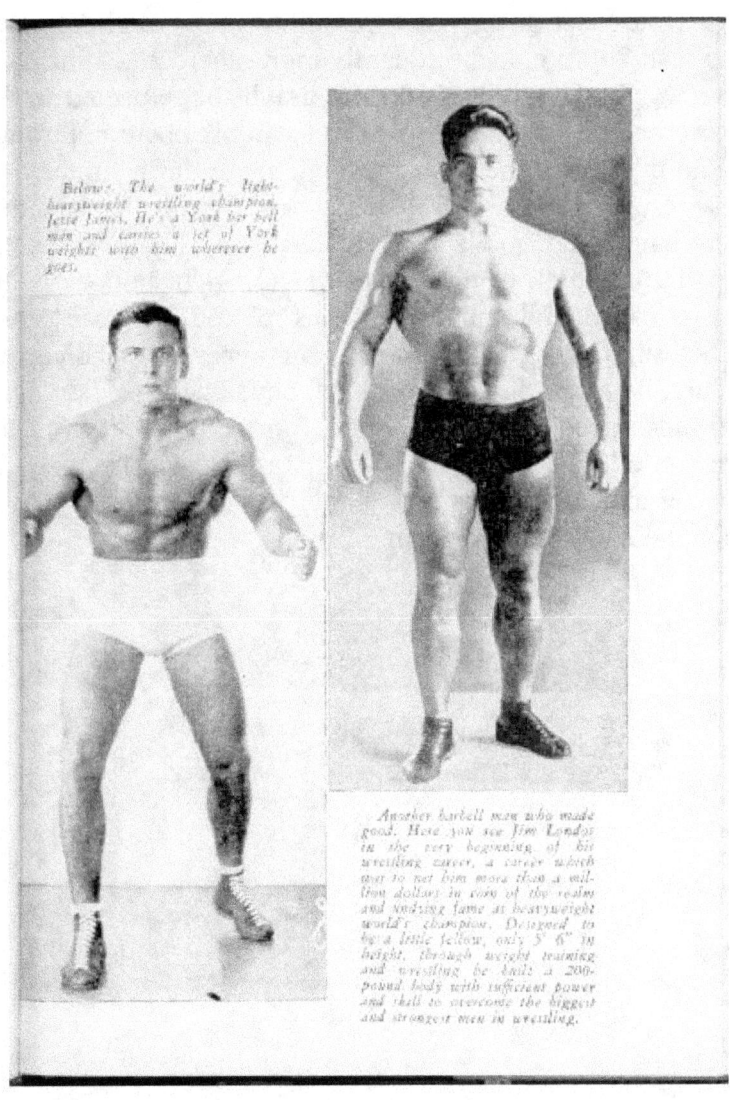

Below: The world's light-heavyweight wrestling champion, Jette Jones. He's a York bar bell man and carries a lot of York weights with him wherever he goes.

Another barbell man who made good. Here you see Jim London in the very beginning of his wrestling career, a career which that to net him more than a million dollars in coin of the realm and undying fame as heavyweight world's champion. Designed to be a little fellow, only 5' 6" in height, through weight training and wrestling he built a 200-pound body with sufficient power and skill to overcome the biggest and strongest men in wrestling.

In football usually the bigger man has the advantage, but there are exceptions to all rules: the good little man, who outplays the pretty good big fellows. In the last few years if you carefully read the statistics of those who have been selected as Ail-American football players, you have noted that while most of them are big fellows not weighing much less than 200 pounds, frequently more, there are some stars who weigh as little as 150. This might be expected in the quarterback post where a man can win his position through the ability to call the plays, through his gridiron strategy, or as a result of his ability to pass or run with the ball, but there have been small men who have won line positions in big time football. One of these was O'Brien, famous Notre Dame 155-pound guard. He was placed on many Ail-American teams. Starting with an apparent handicap in stature, he made the most of it and developed such strength, skill and speed that he not only won the position from the many good men in his school but was selected from scores of thousands of guards throughout the nation to be placed upon the All-American team.

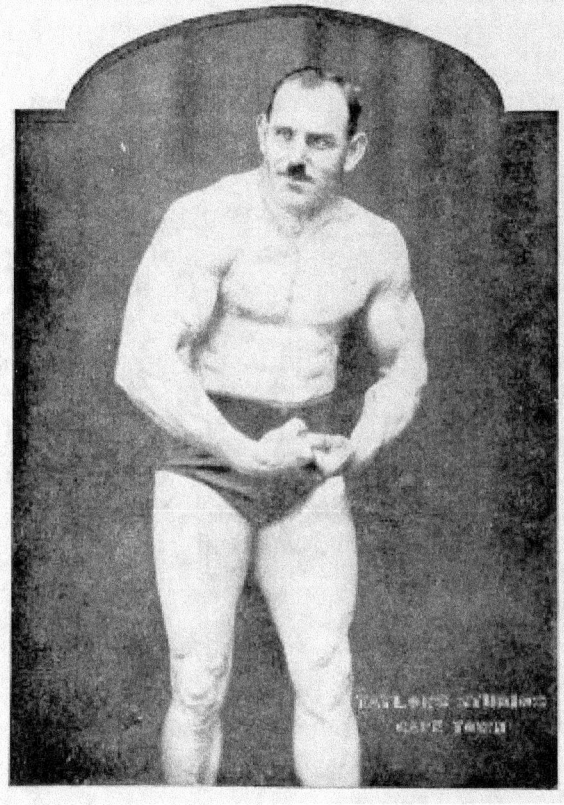

In rowing there have been some good little men, men who have weighed 150 or even 160 and have managed to make the varsity crew. But ordinarily these men are placed in the 150-pound crew, and never does the 150-pound crew defeat the best heavyweight crews. There are many instances where they have beaten the big crew from their own college but they never win at Poughkeepsie, at Philadelphia, or in any of the big regattas. The added weight and power of the big oarsmen is too much for them to overcome. Some light men have rowed in world's and Olympic championship doubles shells, but there is always a stroke of enough power to aid in the winning of this victory. The best scullers are never small fellows. Usually the bigger men sweep the river in the singles event. The world's champion of 1920 and 1924, Jack Kelly, was over six feet tall as is Joe Burke, present world's champion. Yet we must remember that Al Voight, one of my former crewmates at the Vesper Boat Club in Philadelphia, was a short man, although he did develop his body to 168 pounds of muscle. He has been victor in national rowing events, particularly the quarter mile.

There have been some good little men in tennis, but usually the nation's best player, and the world's best player, is a tall man of the six-foot class or more. He has certain advantages in reach, leverage, and power that the little man can seldom overcome. One of the men who brought the Davis cup back to America some years ago was Bill Tilden, six feet two in height. The other was little Bill McLaughlin, scarcely more than five feet two.

In weight throwing the best men are usually big fellows, well over six feet and over 200 pounds in body weight. Blozis of Georgetown, who has been establishing records at shot putting this year, is over six feet and a big, powerful fellow.

Torrence, who established the world's record back in 1935 was a huge man weighing all of 265 pounds, and over six feet in height. I came to know him fairly well on the Olympic trip. He depended too much on his weight and power, not enough on training and skill, and at the Olympics he was defeated by the much smaller, but well trained and Hitler-inspired German weight thrower, Woelke, and failed to even place in the final events. This business of weight throwing is one place where a good big

120

man really excels the good little men. But there have been many small or only average-sized men who have won the varsity positions on the track team through their special training and shot putting ability. Jack Merchant of California of a few years ago was a man who was naturally small, but he developed such great muscular power that he excelled at all weight throwing and was a member of the Olympic team. The really big fellows have ordinarily won this event year after year. Years ago, Ralph Rose, who was a big fat fellow, won the Olympic title with a heave of little more than fifty feet, hardly enough to win in third class competition in this nation today. The marks in other events, as in weight lifting, are ever rising.

In the line of strength there are some events where the little fellows have natural advantages. Usually the best wrist turners are smaller, powerfully built men. They have more favorable turning leverage and often best the really big fellows. Smaller men have advantages in deep knee bending—more favorable leverage. I have seen a little short-legged fellow, only five feet four in height, who succeeded with a deep knee bend of 300 pounds the first time he ever tried it, and Gregory George, commonly called the St. Louis Samson, who trained with us for several months in York, performed a dead weight lift with 600 pounds and a deep knee bend with 400 pounds the first time he ever tried. He had natural advantages of pressing leverage both in arms and legs, was short, not over five feet six, and when he was eleven years of age weighed over 300 pounds. In the last year he usually entered competition at about 260 pounds. Yet these men who are apparently favorably endowed with leg leverage do not hold the deep knee bend records. Henry Steinborn, the famous professional wrestler, a man who weighed 215 pounds at his best, ranks well up among the best deep knee benders of all times. Many years ago in Germany he succeeded with 552 pounds, and he has performed repetitions with 500 pounds. John Davis does not specialize in the deep knee bend but he does well over 500 pounds as does Louis Abele who includes this particular lift regularly in his training.

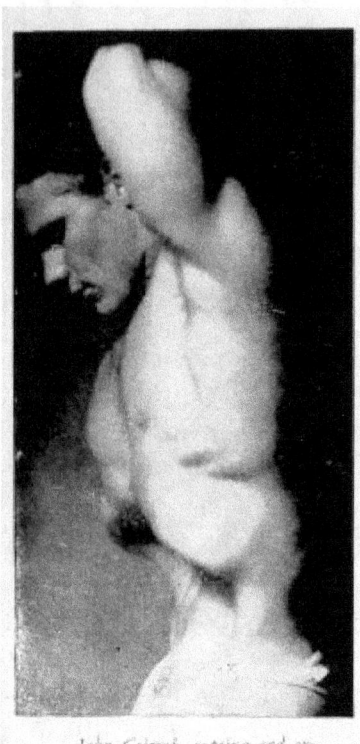

John Grimek, copying and excelling a pose by Ringling Circus's "man without a stomach."

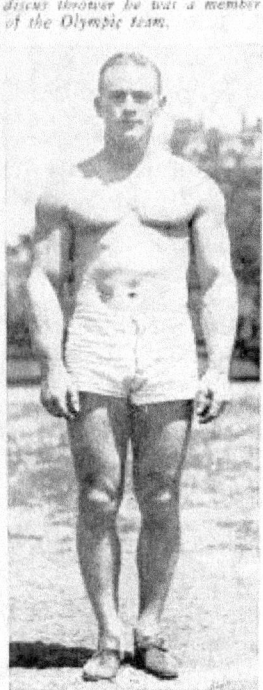

Jack Merchant of California, a weight throwing star of a few years ago. As a shot putter and discus thrower he was a member of the Olympic team.

Do you see what I am getting at? That a good big man is always better than a good little man. That you will be better by increasing your weight and power. Weight is controlled by the body framework and if you train properly you will never become so heavy that you will be considered to be overweight. There is only one man I know who thinks at times that he has too much muscle, and that one man is John Grimek. He puts on weight easily although he does retain his narrow waist even when weighing as much as 230, as he did coming back from the Berlin Olympics. At that body weight he was the huskiest individual I have ever seen. He controls his weight very well and a year later, deciding to enter the 181-pound class in national competition, he reduced his weight and scaled just 176. He had reduced his weight fifty-four pounds. He very easily gets tremendous muscles and endeavors to hold his weight at about 190, at which he believes that he looks better, and I agree with him. But there is only one Grimek. I don't know anyone else who is able to develop too much muscle.

In some quarters added weight is the prime desire; but weight without pleasing proportions and the strength to go with it is not desirable. While there is real beauty in the curves of a well-developed man's muscles, the curves of a fat man's body and limbs are actually repugnant. And while the fat man develops some strength—he must have some to carry his huge body around—he cannot be fast and really powerful. His muscles are not trained to act speedily and powerfully, for to apply power, weight and strength, skill, speed and balance are required by the athlete.

Skill and balance are tremendous factors in athletics today. At first thought one might think that no lighter man would have any chance against a bigger, heavier man, but there are a great many men as we have been discussing who have acquired such quality of muscle, such speed and nervous energy, such balance and skill that they are more than a match for the bigger, heavier men. So don't be discouraged if you are slight in stature and short in height; thousands of other men have shown the way and reached a high position in the world of strength and development.

There are numberless cases of men of short stature who have become unbelievably strong by developing their physical qualities.

My friend John Y. Smith enjoyed training with dumbells and one of his favorite feats was to walk a distance of two blocks carrying a 200-pound dumbell in each hand. He never weighed more than 168 pounds at any stage of his life, and did not look nearly that heavy. The story is told that one day he was passing a group of workmen who were laboring and growling about the hardness of their task as they carried 100-pound sacks of cement one at a time. John Y. stopped for a moment and laughingly said to one of the men, "What's so heavy about the work you are doing that you are eternally kicking?" One of them paused and said, "These sacks are darned heavy. I'll bet you can't even lift one, let alone carry it up that runway and into the concrete mixer. Take off your coat and see if you can lift one." Without removing his coat, Smith swung one to shoulder height with one hand, then pressed it to arm's length overhead, bent press style; after that he reached down for another sack in "two hands anyhow style," and walked into the building carrying these two sacks of cement. You can be sure that an astonished group of workmen gazed at him in respect and wondered how in the world a man could be so strong.

When I see a man perform a feat of strength it gives me real pleasure. Consider a man like Wally Zagurski. Wally is five feet six in height—less than average—not particularly big boned, was a member of the 1932 Olympic team and competed in the 148-pound class. A year later he was 165-pound senior national champion; in fact that year he won five weight lifting championships—all there were. He later competed in the 181-pound class, and two years later missed the 181 title simply because he started too high in one lift, had been in a car smashup the night before and didn't realize that this would handicap his lifting.

Starting with an average frame and light bones, he has become so strong that one day recently I saw him easily and perfectly bent press to arm's length the great weight of 300 pounds, not once but several times. Wally has difficulty locking his arm under a heavy press, but he puts them up there with ridiculous ease. It was the first time I saw 300 pounds held in one hand and pushed to arm's length, and I was thrilled beyond words. Wally constantly surprises all members of the York team with his unusual feats of strength. One of these feats is to pile up, grasp and balance five assorted dumbells, and put them up with one hand.

I could go on telling stories like this indefinitely, for there are so many to illustrate my point, but pages fill up rapidly, books aren't so big, and I must constantly hold myself back in the telling of too many tales. But I want to impress one point upon your mind: that, regardless of your height, your type of bones, your ancestry, your health, with proper training you can become an exceptional physical specimen and win for yourself much honor and glory through your admiration-creating physique, your symmetry, muscular development and strength.

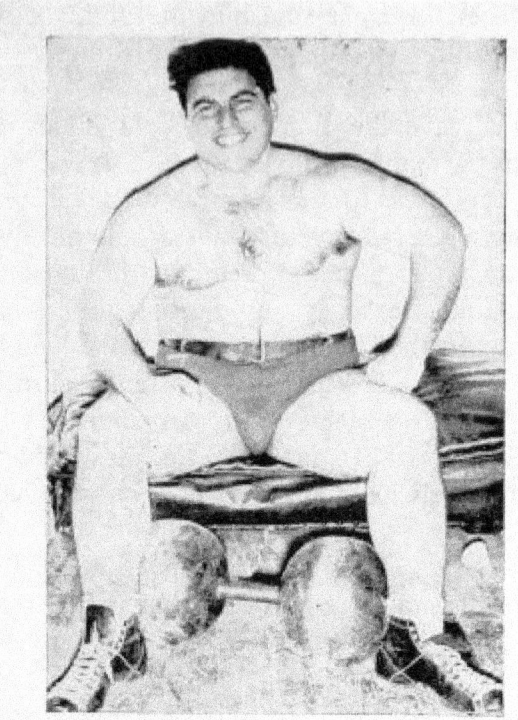

Good-natured Gregory George, the St. Louis Sampson.

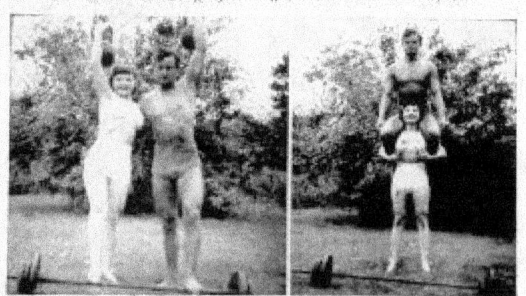

Harold Paden of Akron, O., and Gracie Bard, training at Gracie's home.

CHAPTER SEVEN
Development of Muscle as a Means to Strength and Perfect Proportions

There is a tremendous and widespread interest in physical development. Hardly a man who at some stage of his career, in boyhood, as a youth, or in early manhood who does not wish to be stronger and better developed. Hardly one of us who at some time has not pictured himself as a strong, athletic man. It is estimated that over a million men are following with greater or lesser regularity my system of progressive training. I do not mention this to repeat that I have grown in popularity and been given the privilege to guide the physical endeavors of so many hundreds of thousands of people, but just to emphasize again the widespread interest in the acquisition of physical strength and development.

Only a fraction of those who aspire are willing to perspire, to persist. Many follow the wrong methods, training ideas which seem easier, and thus do not reach their goal at the end of the road to superhealth, strength and development. Some of these who are at first misinformed, wrongly led, persist, find that progressive exercise, constantly striving to handle more and more weight, is the proper road and in the end are successful. It is these enthusiastic or perhaps persistent men and women to whom I am directing the message this book contains. I cannot repeat too often that regardless of starting strength or condition, regardless of age and the life one has led, great beneficial results will be obtained through progressive exercise.

Naturally those who have neglected their physical selves for many long years will find the early conditioning, the handling of light weights, to require a bit more time before they show noticeable progress than will the man who is already fairly strong and healthy, the result of the life he has led, who can plunge in and make rapid progress from the beginning. It is essential that a man have real interest, that he be enthusiastic, that he sincerely desire to gain, that he be willing to put forth reasonable effort. Any teacher will tell you that the pupils who are interested, who really enjoy their studies, will learn more quickly and in the end know vastly more about a subject than will the pupils who dislike what they are studying.

Similarly the person who sincerely enjoys physical training, who can build enthusiasm, will gain most in the end. But even if one should loathe, dislike, hate, detest and abhor physical training, if he will persist he will benefit in the end, for progressive training is the best form of insurance one could obtain to guarantee a long, useful and healthy life with a full share of health, strength and development. I am sure that you will come to enjoy a form of exercise as interesting as weight or cable training and weight lifting.

I have been seeking to prove to you in chapter after chapter that you need not be a fatalist about your body—— believe if you are twenty-five or thirty-five or forty-five that you cannot make satisfactory gains; that you will always be thin and scrawny since you are that way now and your ancestors before you have been in that condition. While heredity governs your physical self to a certain extent, most of heredity is living habits. Some people think that their fatness or thinness runs in the family, but it is usually habits of eating or living that run in the family. If you are one of this sort, do not think that strength and development just happen. They are something that you must work for. I am offering you the easiest, quickest and most result-producing method of training, and you can profit by it if you will but persist in your endeavor.

I know many brothers who are strong men. The Nordquest brothers have been mentioned. Wally Zagurski has been mentioned, but nothing has been said of the fact that he has a brother larger and stronger naturally than Wally. Tony Zagurski was better endowed by nature than Wally; a few years ago when I saw him at Los Angeles, he could perform a stiff-legged dead weight lift with 600 pounds. He paid us a visit recently, the first in eight years, and I was surprised at the strength he possesses. Wally, on the other hand, had to work for what he possesses.

Steve Stanko has a brother who seems to be even more favorably endowed by nature, yet is not interested enough to train. Steve is twice as strong as this brother. Tony Terlazzo has several brothers—one is the second best middleweight in the nation, second to our own national and world's champion middleweight, Johnny Terpak—yet Tony has other brothers who are not interested and never will have the great strength of him and his brother John, particularly the older brother who had to go to work early in life to help support the large and growing family of little Terlazzos. One would never dream that he was a brother of the great York lifter. This was solely an example of intense interest, persistence, physical ambition materializing into winning for this small man, frail in the beginning, the title of " world's best weight lifter."

Johnny Terpak has a brother about the same in size and appearance, who is not so interested and lifts 300 pounds less. It was special training that accounted for this difference. Both had the same advantages of heredity and the same mode of living. Up in Rochester, New York, there are two sets of brothers, the younger of whom in both families appears destined to gain more renown than his elder brothers. The first of these are the two brothers of the Tanney family. The elder Tanney was a pretty good weight lifter a few years back. He had a younger brother whose photos appear in the "Road to Super Strength" as an ordinary lad of thirteen just starting bar bell training and at fifteen as a really husky fellow well on the way to becoming a weight lifting champion. Armand now at eighteen lifts 320 pounds overhead, is not only much larger and stronger than his elder brother but any other member of his immediate family. Frank Carbone was the elder brother in the other family. Although small and slight in the beginning, he became interested in physical betterment through weight lifting, and has built a very nice and really powerful physique. On several occasions he has been lifting champion in his body weight class in western New York. The next brother, August, had a very poor beginning; at fifteen he looked like some underprivileged young man who had never had any of the advantages of life. But at sixteen what a trans-formation! One would hardly know that he was the same man. You can judge by the photo which appears in this book. And now there is another Carbone.

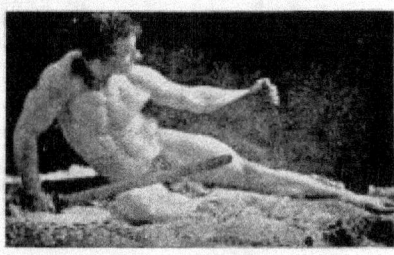

Eugene Sandow.

The "before" picture he offers shows what a poor start he had; the "now" picture shows a similar remarkable transformation as compared to the great improvement brother August made. He is not only larger than either of his brothers but vastly stronger; he can lift a great deal more than either of them and is the weight lifting champion in his class. Here we have three young Carbones who certainly weren't much physically to begin with, but every

130

one of them through progressive training with weights and weight lifting has built strength, muscles and bodily symmetry of which he can be proud. I could go on and on, using reams of paper, writing a book several times this size with a never-ending stream of physical successes the result of following these "proven to be best" methods about which I am writing. Surely you are becoming convinced and feel that you would like to go and do likewise. It is not natural advantages, bone size, or luck which brought these young men I have listed to the top; it was persistent efforts with training methods such as I am offering here.

So many parents believe that the young man does not need special exercise. They think that hard work and play in the earlier years will be sufficient. Millions of people live in this country who played when they were young and worked when they became older, who are thin, fat, weak, sick, ailing, caricatures of what humans should be. Play, athletic sports and games are admirable, but they are not the best form of physical training. Too often the weak boy or girl does not have the opportunity to play, for even in childhood when teams are chosen, everyone wants to play on the side with the best players, and the boys or girls who lack ability are left out. And later in life when high school and college are reached, even where there is compulsory physical training, the underdeveloped manage to slide by while neglecting their physical selves, just going through the motions of physical exercise. Just as some people can graduate from school and know very little and others can lead their classes, seventy per cent is sufficient for graduation, but seventy per cent of physical efficiency is nothing to be proud of, and is far from a satisfactory rating to fight the battle of life.

Setting up exercises at school or in the army are better than nothing, but individual training with proper personal instruction is the way to physical perfection. Glass drills offer little benefit. The more athletic, stronger and more enduring members of the class are held back by the weaker members. Exercises which might cause a business man sadly out of condition to puff and pant and feel that he had a workout would be nothing for the powerful men of the York Bar Bell Club. The individual during such training learns little if anything of his own capacity for bodily improvement.

At schools where athletics are one of the chief interests, there are high-salaried coaches who coach the favored few, but the average individual gets none of it. It is far better for each individual to become sufficiently interested to exercise alone or with a friend, to exercise intelligently, for only in this way is the maximum of benefit obtained.

There are so many young fellows who succeed physically in spite of parental apathy, disinterest or even disapproval. Many men have wives who are not interested, or who may even laugh a little at their training. Parents and wives should encourage. There is no better hobby than physical exercise. There is no better habit. Husbands who have the physical training hobby are wholesome, healthy, happy, contented men. They build up strength, energy, superhealth, have placid dispositions, are good company and are destined for success. Far better for the husband or the son to be interested in physical training than to shoot pool, gamble, play cards, hang around the corner, or even "chase" other men's wives. When I meet a wife or parents who at times complain about the noise friend husband or son makes, I tell them that they are very lucky to have a man in the family, young or old, who makes a fetish of muscular development; it's the best hobby of all.

There is little change in the fashions as far as men's bodies are concerned. Women strove for the wine glass effect in the last century, later they were admired for their well-upholstered appearance, and so many women wore bustles, false breasts and even wrapped bandages around their calves to make them larger. Next there was the round-shouldered, flat-chested, bent-backed, flapper type of girl who walked with bent knees and a curve in her back. And still later there was a liking for the athletic, well-developed type of girl, and fortunately that is the trend at present.

But the well-developed man of 2,500 years ago if he could come back to life in his prime would look well in the tailored suits of today, and if our best-built men were back in the year of 600 b.c., they could easily pose for the statues of the day. Men's physiques don't change. Broad shoulders, sturdy necks, big round chests, thick arms, and powerful legs were always admired and they always will be admired. The styles in clothes change slightly, but the well-developed, symmetrical male physique is always the subject of much admiration and favorable comment.

Every day I receive a great many letters from those who are following my training methods and from others who are contemplating following a good bar bell system. Some say they will take my course if I can guarantee that they will gain twenty pounds in five months' time. Another will write that he will take my course of training if I will make him twice as strong in a few months' time. I tell the first man that I cannot guarantee the gain of a pound a week for twenty weeks, for I cannot control his life or his habits. And I tell him of many who have gained tremendously, just as I am relating tales of a few of them in the chapters of this book. I tell him that I have every confidence that he can increase the size or circumference of his chest by five inches in five months' time, that he can increase the size of his arm two inches in that period and his neck two and a half inches. And right there he may say, " But I don't want a neck that big. I want to be strong and well built but I don't want to be too big." And there we strike our first stumbling block, for a man cannot be made several times as strong without being bigger, nor can he expect to build his shoulders and his arms but not his legs or his neck. All are parts of the same body, all are served by the same internal system, and when one part benefits the other sections of the body attain like advantages.

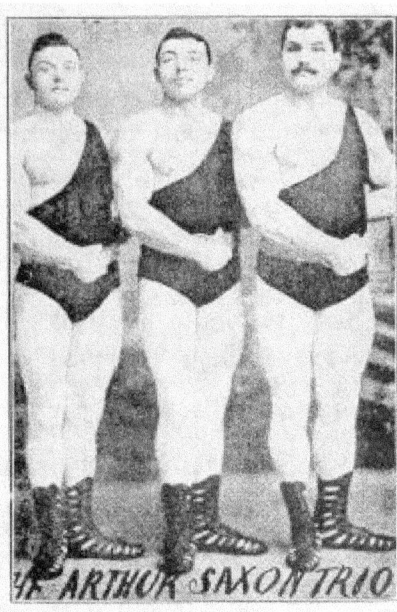

The famous Saxon trio. Left to right: Herman, Curt and Arthur. While Arthur was the largest and by far the strongest, the others were tremendously powerful, too.

It may surprise a man who wears a thirteen and a half collar to know that he will need a size sixteen in a few months, and that if he has been wearing a size thirty-six coat he will need a forty-four in a few months—that he will need to have first altered and then replaced all of his clothing except perhaps his pocket handkerchiefs and his neckties. It does seem at first that such a change will be abrupt and

134

fortunately there are not many who are concerned about becoming too big. The majority wishes to become bigger; that's why they are interested in physical training. I can usually satisfy the doubts of these men by showing them others who have the forty-four-inch chests they will acquire and the sixteen-inch arms.

If I were talking to a beginner and would tell him that in a few years his thirty-five-inch chest should increase to forty-eight, his twelve-inch arm to seventeen and a half, his thirteen-inch neck to eighteen, he would hardly believe me and would no doubt feel that he wouldn't want to have measurements that large. So many of them have asked, "Bob, how much should I weigh at my height of five feet eight?" I point out various members of our team, if it is our training time, which is the usual period when I do most of my talking with visitors. I do much of my writing at home. I am away a lot, but I try to be at the gymnasium at training time as often as possible. I can help the hard-training, ambitious members of our team quite a bit and perhaps get in a little training myself. So I have plenty of illustrations to give to my interrogators. "You will weigh from 180 to 200 pounds," is my reply. "I wouldn't want to be that heavy," they will say. "Why not?" is my usual comeback. "See Wally Zagurski over there; he weighs 180 at his height of five feet six. Wouldn't you like to have his superb development?" The answer is always in the affirmative. "And there's the great John Grimek; he weighs just under 200, is approximately your height. Wouldn't you like to have a body like his?" "You're darn right I would," is usually the reply. "It's his pictures more than any other one thing that has interested me in physical training."

135

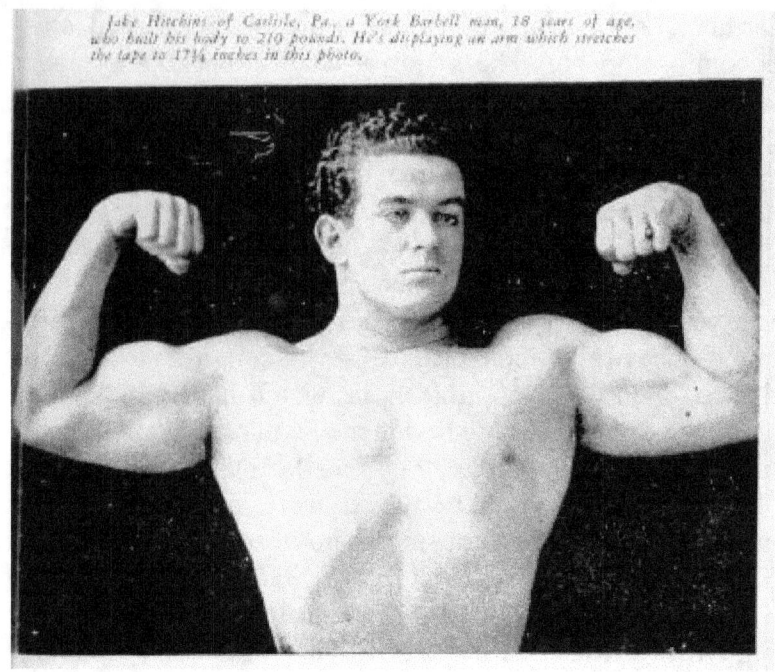

It is really surprising that so few people know anything about their bodies. They seem to take everything for granted, know nothing of their physical possibilities. I can understand how a man can wear the same watch for many years or drive the same car without knowing what goes on inside or beneath the hood but I can't quite imagine a person living with his body for so many years and knowing nothing about it. The other day a visitor asked me what I weigh at present. "Two hundred and sixty," I replied. I have weighed 265 and my weight fluctuates a bit depending upon my training or my mode of living at the particular time. I gain when I train more intensively and lose a bit when I am less active. With most people it is the opposite, but muscles weigh more than fat and when I train hard I get more muscle. My new friend said, "Two hundred and sixty? I wouldn't want to carry all that weight around with me." "I don't carry it around," I said. "It carries me— easily, effortlessly and tirelessly." I feel like I weigh a hundred pounds instead of 260, I'm so light on my feet. It is only when a man or woman carries a big tub of fat around at the waistline and carries spare tires and paddings of fat over all the body that it is necessary to carry the weight around. But muscle, half the muscular bulk of the body in the legs, carries the man, and my weight carries me around.

Regardless of a man's physical desires—to gain weight, lose weight, improve athletic ability so that he can make the school team or beat his friends at golf—whether he is past the age of maturity, past middle age, or really old, he can obtain his physical desires by application of the proper training methods.

We have well-built strong men of all sizes and types. The little fellows of the Firpo Lemma height, men who are dwarf-like in their construction, less than five feet tall, have gained nicely. Firpo is ideally built with a weight of 123 pounds at his height of four feet ten. At five feet two we find that the ideal body weight for men like Art Levan and Dick Bachtell is 132. Art is heavier for he has developed amazing strength and lifting ability. The next step upward finds Tony Terlazzo, height five feet four at 148 pounds. Two more inches and we have five feet six, the ideal weight of a well-developed man of Johnny Terpak's height being 165. At five feet eight we find Johnny Davis, looking beautifully built at 181. Johnny weighs more now for he is so phenomenal but he displayed a most attractive physique when he weighed 181. At six feet we have Steve Stanko; the correct weight for this height according to my chart of height and weight for the heavy-boned is 213, just a bit lighter than Stanko's Herculean build.

Depending upon your type of bone construction, you can build a symmetrical body which will approximate these weights. If you are a very small man you will know that your thirteen-inch arm in the case of little Firpo will become strong enough to press a great weight, 210 in his case, deep knee bend with 300. If you are five feet two you will know that you can win a fourteen-inch arm, and this fourteen-inch arm, like the thirteen-inch arm of Firpo, will have such fine proportions that it will look just like the eighteen-inch arm of Grimek and Stanko. If you are five feet four you are getting in the sixteen-inch arm class when very well developed, and at five feet six you will be taller, but cannot expect much greater measurements than the 148-pounder. Most men when well developed weigh in these classes, the 148 and the 165, and there is usually little difference between the 148 and the 165 in chest measurement or in arm measurement. The difference in weight is invariably due to the difference in height. When you are five feet eight, immediately you attain the possibilities of a forty-eight-inch chest and a sixteen-and-a- half-inch arm. Grimek's arm at that weight is more than seventeen inches; John Davis's arm, approximately sixteen and a half. Wally Zagurski's arm is seventeen inches. But when you reach the six foot mark, you can build a chest of fifty inches or more.

Whether you are tall or short, whether as short as the five foot two members of our team or as tall as the six foot four and a half Jack Cooper, you will attain similar proportions. You will attain measurements which will accentuate the beautiful lines of your figure. You can be fast, graceful in appearance and will never be slow or clumsy regardless of how much muscle you pack onto that frame of yours.

When a man is of the light-boned type, he can add thirty or forty pounds to his physique and still be comparatively slender. Take my own case again: Whether at 260 or 265 I am almost slender. Legs and arms are big, chest is deep, shoulders fairly broad, but I am bony around the collarbone, the ribs; my face is thin, my waist fourteen inches smaller than my chest, and altogether I look athletic and slender. If I weighed less I would merely look undeveloped. It is surprising how much weight and muscle your frame requires to cover it.

Most young men have about as little muscular development as is essential to carry them around and permit them to go about their daily living. If such a man is of average height he would weigh perhaps 130 to 140 pounds. What a transformation when that man starts to train and gains weight and muscle. He should put on forty pounds, and when he is well developed, what a beautifully moulded specimen of humanity he will be. Such a young man, if he follows the rules of living as well as of proper training, will grow so rapidly that you can almost see him pack on the pounds and the inches of muscle.

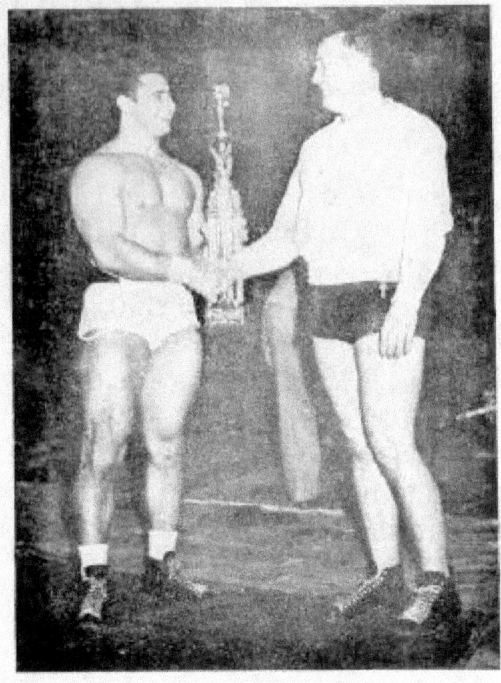

CHAPTER EIGHT
Strength Through Symmetrical Development

Of the many desirable physical qualities, strength, power, weight, big muscles, quality of muscle, symmetry, I list the latter first, and I am ably seconded in my preference by the majority of leaders in the world of strength and development. I believe that if a census could be taken of the ambitious body builders of the nation, we would find that ninety-five per cent of them would prefer a symmetrical body to one that is just big or even powerful.

Symmetry of physique is one thing the average public understands. While many people believed that Eugene Sandow was the strongest man in the world, the majority knew and admired him solely for his symmetrical physique. Sandow weighed approximately 180 pounds during his career and although he was very strong for his weight there have been scores of men since he first acquired fame who are stronger. Few of them are known to the public, but everyone knows Sandow, and it was his splendid physique which built this undying renown for him.

Flo Ziegfeld, who attained great fame for glorifying the American girl in his perennial series of Ziegfeld Follies, made his start glorifying the male physique in the person of Eugene Sandow. These two men teamed up when Sandow was demonstrating his strength in the dime museums of New York. They reached the heights together with Sandow touring the nation and later the world with a strength and muscle control act. Few of the millions of people who were fortunate enough to see Sandow in action at the peak of his career can remember what he did in the way of strength feats but none of them has forgotten or will ever forget his muscle posing act. Sandow had blond curly hair, and the contrast of his splendid body with the black background of

141

his posing cabinet, with the bright light overhead, made him immortal. Of course Sandow deserved all the credit which came his way, for he built this physique, studied anatomy, his own good points and his weak spots, made the most of his bony framework and made a masterpiece of his body.

Many development enthusiasts believe Sandow to have been the best-built man of the modern world. His physique was more highly publicized than any of his contemporaries', so some of the other marvelously built men of his time are little known. In the beginning of Sandow's career a number of strong men were claiming to be the world's strongest men. Cyclops, Washington Irving, Apollon and, later, Louis Cyr and Arthur Saxon were the best known of these men. They all considered strength of paramount importance, cared little for the appearance of their physiques and the majority of them are completely forgotten at present. Sandow was really strong, athletic, and a good showman. This, coupled with a splendid physique, made him famous. Bobby Pandour showed more muscular definition, more exceptional development and, judging by the photos we have seen of him, he had a beautiful, symmetrical physique. Yet he is hardly known. He lacked either showmanship or the proper publicity.

Before going on with our discussion, it is interesting to contemplate whether Eugene Sandow or John Grimek, the best-built man of the present, has the better physique. Opinions will be divided and it will be just as difficult to choose between them as it is at present to settle the arguments about whether Jim Jeffries could beat Gene Tunney, or whether Jack Johnson was not a better all-around fighter than Joe Louis, or whether the raging, tearing, swinging, fighting machine, old John L. Sullivan, could not have defeated Jack Dempsey at his best. Impossible to bring them together at one time and to make the necessary comparison.

All we have of Sandow is a great many photos to illustrate his physique. Many of these photos are beautiful, most are above average, but some are quite bad. Most of the latter are little known but they are in existence. It was never my pleasure to see Sandow in the flesh, but I do see a great deal of John Grimek and have over a period of years. And he is one man who looks much more outstanding in person than in his marvelous photos. His photos possess considerable originality and more life, action or rhythm than the Sandow poses. I have never seen a bad or even a poor picture of Grimek. From every position, whether clothed or training in the gym, from any angle, he presents a splendid picture. Grimek is considerably stronger than Sandow ever was. Of course he weighs more, normally nearly twenty pounds more, and as a result has a more Herculean development. Grimek's presses of over 300 pounds, his great power in any sort of strength feat, his lifting ability, all stamp him as a real strong man. Grimek cares much more for development than for lifting or even strength feats, but he has resented at times that others have said approximately as follows, "Now that he has the muscles, what can he do with them?" "He's muscle bound: probably can't even touch the back of his neck, his arms are so big." So John had to spend a little time at strength feats, lifting of weights, winning of championships; he has been senior national lifting champion in the heavyweight class, made the highest lifting records of any American at the Olympic games of 1936, won the championships of North America, lifted in Vienna as a member of the world's championship team. Cleaning and pressing two dumbells, one weighing 125, the other 110, well illustrate his strength. He's a product of the slogan, "Train for shape and strength

143

is sure to follow." He learned that very heavy exercises bring best results.

Heavy weights in the exercises have been responsible for most of the great Grimek physique. But this is not all: he has practiced an all-around program consisting of "the thousand exercises," has made a study of his physique, brought out its good points and eliminated its bad ones.

Years ago he was quite ordinary in development. In a comparatively short time he built himself to a husky 175 pounder and commenced to obtain some renown for his development. In those early days I was not impressed with his physique; he was long-waisted and broad-waisted, he looked short in the legs, and did not have the clear-cut definition of muscles he now possesses. Scientific, progressive training moulded his physique to its present symmetrical proportions.

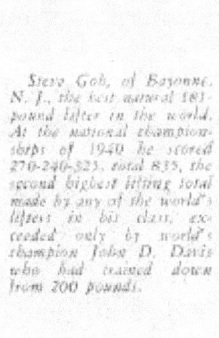
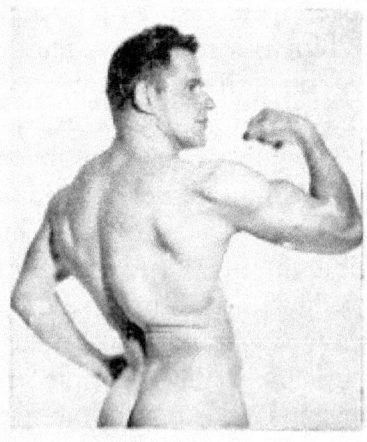

Steve Gob, of Bayonne, N. J., the best amateur 181-pound lifter in the world. At the national championships of 1940 he scored 270-240-325, total 835, the second highest lifting total made by any of the world's lifters in his class, exceeded only by world's champion John D. Davis who had trained down from 200 pounds.

John Grimek, unlike Topsy, did not just grow. It took long and hard work; hours a day of training in the beginning, nearly every day in the week. But now that he has the physique he trains less than any man I know. One of the New York City columnists, in writing about Grimek, said that he must spend hours and hours each day training, that he must go to bed early, have ten or twelve hours of sleep, watch his diet very carefully and live a life of privation and application to his muscle building which prevents him from having any pleasure. This rigid training program is necessary for a man who is training for a championship fight, for an oarsman who will row with his crew at Poughkeepsie, for a runner, but not for a weight lifter.

Grimek trains in what might be called spasms. It is really a glorified method of irregular training which will be discussed later. He does not train for a considerable period and then he comes into the gym and trains very intensively, using extremely heavy weights and practicing a wide variety of exercises. This gave rise to the tale which appeared among other stories in the liars' competition in Strength and Health magazine, that all one need do to obtain a physique like Grimek is to train like he does, particularly use the weights he handles in every exercise. The story went that, if you take 320 pounds and perform ten presses with it, 500 pounds and perform fifteen deep knee bends, the same weight and go through a routine of dead weight lifting exercises, you will build arms, legs, shoulders, back and chest like Grimek's. But this does not account for the wasplike waist of Grimek, wasp-like in comparison with the remainder of his body. It was suggested that all one need do is go to a hospital, make an appointment with a good surgeon and have about thirty feet of intestine removed and the slender waist would result. The writer of this system of training admitted that he had not tried this method, but had every confidence that it would work.

Joking aside, we do have in our midst today a man whom we believe to be a better all-around physical specimen, with Herculean strength and near-perfect proportions, than any man who has flashed across the strong man firmament in the past, or who exists in the present. It may be many long years before a man who has the Grimek combination of strength and development will come forward. While all of us with similar training methods as compared to those employed by Grimek will greatly improve our physiques, there is only one Grimek and most of us cannot hope to have such a physique. Frequently the friends of a certain strength athlete who have never seen Grimek, hail their friend as another Grimek. Many strength athletes learn to pose well and show their physiques to the best advantage in photos, and are frequently disappointing when you see them in person. But Grimek is always outstanding. He is a splendid example for us to follow in our endeavors to build exceptional physiques.

Symmetry of physique means balance of all the parts. And this symmetry which is so pleasing to the eye is balance as we see it rather than the results as shown by the tape measure. Although the artists believe that a symmetrical body is one in which the biceps, calf and neck are identical in size, such a man very likely would not appear symmetrical to the eye. Largest measurement of the neck, next largest measurement the calf, with the arm measurement in the last position, will result if proper exercise is followed. By specializing in arm development and neglecting the development of the neck and calf, some men have achieved similar measurements of these parts, but not a symmetrical physique.

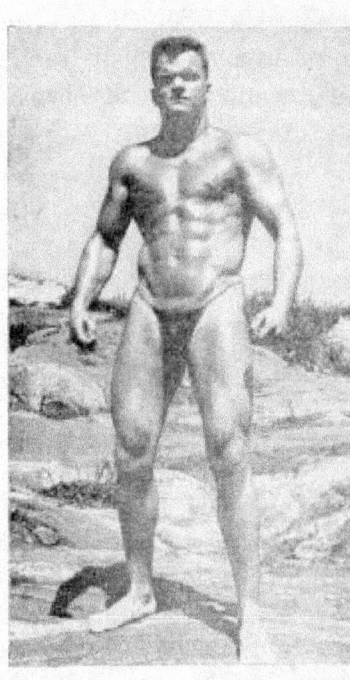

A man cannot have a symmetrical physique if the upper body, including big arms, broad shoulders, deep, well-muscled chest, is carried around by a slender pair of legs, and its opposite counterpart—powerful, well-developed legs with narrow shoulders and an upper body lacking in development—will not be symmetrical. Although absolute symmetry has not been achieved by any man, this perfect development is most clearly approached by the weight lifters of the present who practice an all-around system of training with heavy exercises interspersed with some body-building exercises designed to amplify the strength and development of any parts of their bodies which may be lacking.

A man who has a really symmetrical body invariably, regardless of his height and weight, will have a definite relation of proportions—certain shoulder width in relation to his height; a definite girth of arms and legs in relation to the body, of thighs to that of the hips, and the arms a certain size in comparison with the chest.

We have before us today, as we contemplate the great physiques which have been won by the weight lifting champions, Terry, Terlazzo, Terpak, Davis and Stanko, and with these champions we must include a number of additional men who were place winners in the national championship, who have symmetrical physiques—men like Steve Gob, Dennis Schemanski, Gord Venables, of course Grimek, Frank Dorio, Bernard Baran, Eddie Harrison, Dick Bachtell and so many others, men who prove what has always been a theory of mine, that symmetrical development, balance of the parts of the man's body, equal development in all the parts, is responsible for a large measure of the power of the strong man. Since professional strong acts are no longer in vaudeville, which is hardly in existence itself, we must judge by our amateur competitive lifters who take part in national and international competition.

All of our champions, Terry, Terlazzo, Terpak, Davis and Stanko, are renowned for their physiques, all have won honors for development as well as strength, all are magnificently built, have attained near-perfect bodies, and very great strength, all are the products of all-around training, the practice of a great many exercises, both of a very heavy and fairly light nature, with a great deal of weight lifting practice included in their programs. They in many cases trained for strength, and shapeliness resulted. But if a man who is all out of shape to begin with, who takes up the practice of physical training to improve his body, persists with the progressive system, constantly striving to handle more and more weight, he will obtain better proportions, but vastly greater strength and weight lifting ability, if he chooses to employ his muscles in the lifting of weights. From the very beginning of my professional career, from my rise from a complete unknown to the world's leading physical director, I have laid particular emphasis on this all-around development, this all-around training program. Instead of following only the systems so freely advocated by those who believe that the acquisition of weight and more strength is sufficient, I have urged all the men under my personal direction such as the members of the famous York team, such as my scores of thousands of hard-training pupils, and even the casual readers of Strength and Health magazine, to practice an all-around program consisting of weight lifting exercises and body-building movements— the thousand exercises. And the years have proven, by the way that York-trained athletes lead the world in strength and development, that these training methods are the best. All of these men who tried to become unusually strong became unusually well developed, and all men who strive to become unusually well developed become exceptionally strong. There are a few exceptions to this latter rule: those who neglect their lower bodies or their backs and endeavor to build the perfect physique, practicing only exercises which show up well when training in front of a mirror which reflects only the upper body. Such a physique is lacking in strength and the symmetrical development so much to be desired.

There is, besides the definite relationship in size of the various limbs and the trunk of the body, an interdependence between the various parts of the body. If you were employed at work in some factory, which consisted of performing the same simple movement all day long, day after day, and year after year, if sufficient effort were required, you would obtain a lopsided development unless you practiced a fair measure of exercises during your leisure hours

149

to develop all the parts symmetrically. But if your work was to drive spikes in building a railroad, or to saw and chop down trees, you would be required to call upon all of your muscles, for the swinging of a heavy sledge requires the use of all the muscles of the body, back, arms, shoulders, legs, feet and even the toes. Balance or co-ordination is required in these powerful swinging movements.

Balance, the result of all-around training, and symmetrical development, mark the champion in all lines of physical endeavor and sport. It has long been my contention that a really high-class clean and jerk, such as double body weight for the smaller men, and over 300 pounds for the larger fellows, requires a greater combination of physical attributes than any other one feat in the realm of sport. It takes a combination of strength, skill, timing, nervous energy and sheer athletic ability to make the first terrific effort of pulling the weight to the shoulder, and then almost immediately co-ordinating all muscles and power in a slightly different way, to jerk and hold the weight at arm's length. Every muscle of the body plays its part in the explosive effort to make a really high-class clean and jerk. And the champion is the man who has developed quality of muscle, properly balanced muscular proportions, all-around development and the ability to call upon all of these muscles at one time. The two hands snatch and the clean and jerk, in particular, demonstrate the close connection between strength and symmetry of body or between all- around development and strength.

All-around training, first practicing those exercises which build the muscles in groups and then exercises which involve the action of all of those groups, brings the best results. When you think of as simple a movement as curling a dumbell or chinning, you may feel that the biceps is the only muscle group involved, but many more muscles are brought into play. The deep lying muscles—the Brachialis Anticus and the Coracobrachialis—must play their part, and other muscles of the back and chest are connected to the arm bone and must perform their share of the work. All of these muscles depend upon each other. Symmetrical development of the body will make the strong man, for just as a chain is no stronger than its weakest link, the body will be no stronger than the weakest muscle or muscle group involved in a particular movement. All of the muscles must be developed and by striving for a symmetrical development, practicing a wide variety of exercises—to develop all the muscles—will also develop unusual strength.

Men who have obtained what little development they have through tensing exercises never possess an impressive-looking arm. Such an arm, while it may have a good development of the belly of the muscle, will be lacking in development at the end near the elbow as well as the extremity near the shoulder. Such muscles have very little ability to work with their neighboring muscle groups. The man who exercises with free-hand movements, or the once popular club swinging exercises, or even five-pound dumbells or lighter, cannot expect to obtain much in the way of development. If he were to practice the two hands swing or snatch with these five-pound dumbells, in this latter case swinging the bells well back between the legs and then overhead bending backward, he would obtain some slight benefit from the action of the internal muscles and the massaging of his internal organs, but he could not expect much from such light weights, as the large muscles of the body are so tremendously powerful that light weights cannot bring out their full development. The world's record in the back lift (in which a man bends under a heavily loaded platform and then, by straightening the legs and sustaining the weight with the back, raises it an inch or so from the platform) is 4,300 pounds and it is held by Louis Cyr. In

151

the harness lift, in which the legs also play the chief part but where the weight is suspended from the hips and the shoulders while the body is erect and part of the lifting is done by straightening the arms which are placed upon a rail around the lifting platform, the record weight lifted was 3,600. It is evident that such powerful muscles cannot be developed with light methods.

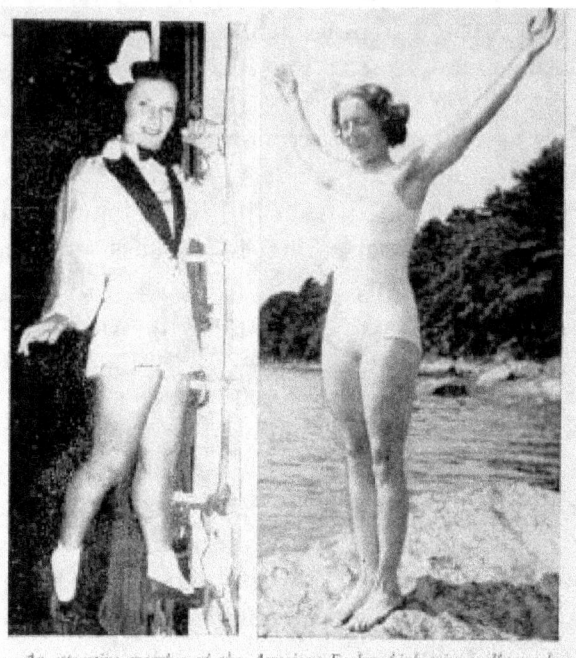

An attractive member of the American Eagles, high wire walkers who demonstrate their ability each year at the Steel Pier in Atlantic City. This little lady is powerful yet presents an appearance that most any girl could envy.

Mrs. Roberta Ranck Bonnewell, best known as "Bobbie" Ranck, during the many years in which she compiled an unequalled string of gymnastic and athletic championships. In 1924 she was crowned as the physically most perfect woman in America. This photo was taken 16 years later. She was all-around gymnastic champion for 16 consecutive years, and has won championships at running, jumping, discus and javelin throwing, fencing and many other sports. Competing against 6,000 competitors in an International Woman's meet at Cologne, Germany, in the pentathlon she won the trophy of victory.

Over a hundred thousand sets of bar bells and dumbells have been shipped by the York Bar Bell Company. These are packed in boxes weighing no, 210, or even 310 pounds.

152

Beyond this two boxes are used. Real strength is required to lift these boxes, to load them upon the trucks which take them to the freight station, and the men who do this work year after year become very powerful in every part of their bodies—so powerful that they can easily toss the boxes in which the adjustable dumbells are packed, a weight of only eighty pounds, to the man who is placing them in position upon the truck. Naturally one could not obtain the strength to do this by light methods. Too often the back, which should be the keystone of a man's strength, is neglected by body builders. They stand in front of the mirror (I think this normally a good idea, for one can more easily see the results obtained, see the muscles which are lacking; it also adds interest to the training program) and exercise only those muscles which can be seen. They neglect in too many cases to exercise the largest and strongest muscles of the body, which must be brought to a high state of development if a man is to become strong or even symmetrically developed. These large muscles of the legs and back must be taught to play their part in the acquisition of strength and development or the maximum of results will not be obtained. All strong men have developed all their muscles or they would not be strong. They would have their weak links and be limited by these weakest parts of their body.

One good way to test the all-around strength of a man, to find if he has a weak link, or an undeveloped part, is to have him lie upon two chairs or two benches in such a way that the head and back of neck are on one chair, the feet on the other. He must be fairly strong to even retain the straightness of the body in this position. If the man is strong enough, put first one man upon his body near the knees, another near the chest and if he is really strong, another across his mid-section. This requires real power and the man who can do it certainly has a strong and symmetrically constructed physique.

153

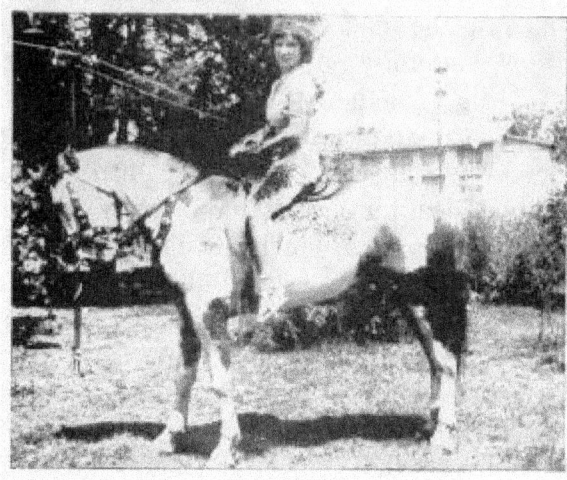

Every muscle from his heels to his head is well developed. This is a feat of pure muscular strength, unlike so many supporting feats—wrestler's bridge, "tomb of Hercules" and others in which a column of bone supports the weight. In this position all the bones are horizontal and only the strength of muscles, tendons and ligaments keeps the body straight. A powerful contraction of the muscles which run from the neck to the base of the spine is required in this common feat of strength. At first thought you may believe that the legs have little to do, because the knees will not bend backward. On the contrary they have a great deal of work to perform, for the muscles on the buttocks and the backs of the legs must exert their maximum force to keep the body straight and to support the weight. You will be impressed with the development of the muscles in the biceps or the back of the legs when the man is once more

154

erect and you can see just how he is put together. The muscles below the hip have just as much work to perform as those above the hip. A star at this feat must be strong all over.

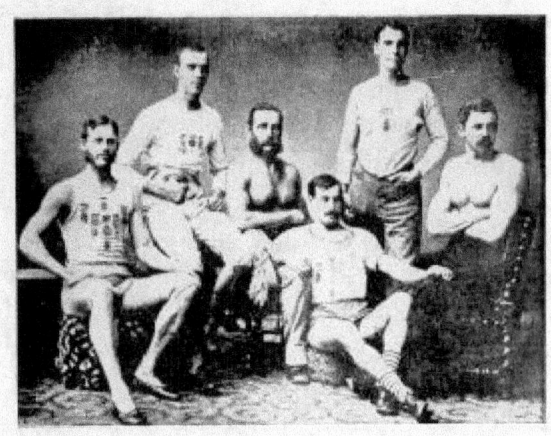

A photo we have long desired to show to the strength-loving public. The original hangs in the great New York Athletic Club of New York City and it nearly required an act of Congress to obtain this copy. Through the efforts of Dietrich Wortmann, national weight-lifting chairman for these many years, and Col. Charles Dieges, both members of the New York Athletic Club and prominent in athletic circles in New York City, former wrestling champions, we finally have the photo. They are the champions of the New York A. C. in 1873. The men shown are Elliott Burns, Geo. I. Baron, W. B. Curtis, Dave M. Stern, Chas. H. Corr, and Harry F. Buermeyer. Father Bill Curtis, the central figure, is our chief interest, for he established world's weight-lifting records before and after the Civil War, some of which still stand. His curl and press of 2,100-pound dumbells while weighing 168 pounds is truly exceptional and his 1250-pound harness lift remains the amateur record.

Very likely you have spent considerable time at bathing beaches and with each passing year the group of strong men, balancers, tumblers and pyramid builders who practice on the beaches grows. Tumblers and balancers must have symmetrical, well-knit frames, and invariably they possess great bodily strength because one cannot tumble without bringing all the muscles of the body into play with resulting development. It is not possible for everyone to practice tumbling; one may not have the inclination, the ability or the place in which to practice. But weight lifting movements can be practiced in any place where there is room to stretch the arms out with a little to spare, seven feet of space being sufficient. Weight lifting repetitions assure all who practice such movements that a symmetrical body, well balanced in strength and proportions, is sure to result.

Before closing this chapter, let us make a close study of the strong man, and since we consider that John Grimek has the greatest combination of strength and development of any man of the present, we will inspect his physique. It is difficult to know where to start, he's so superbly developed; so we will start at the top. Holding his head erect is a big, powerful, muscular, column-like neck. By columnlike I of course mean that the neck is not small at the top, but rises in one muscular column-like mass from the muscles of the shoulders. In the front of this neck there is a clean-cut, muscular appearance of neck and jaw. Following downward we see that the muscles of the neck blend well into the sloping muscles of the shoulders, the trapezius group. If Grimek would raise his shoulders slightly you would observe just how these muscles of the neck blend into those of the shoulders and the upper back. A perfect circle of muscle would appear with a bowl-like deep depression in the center and a ring of powerful, deep-lying muscles around them. These muscles are fully developed for they are the muscles which lift the shoulders or the arms, with anything attached to them, even if it be a 600-pound bar bell. Following the slope of the trapezius muscles to the point of the shoulder we come to a powerful muscle which forms a big cap over the upper arm joint, bearing consid-erable resemblance to a big cocoanut cut in half. The mus-cles of the upper arm blend into the shoulder muscles and in a man like Grimek, a human anatomical chart, you could trace the muscles of the shoulder almost to their point of attachment upon the back of the upper arm bone.

Dropping below the shoulders on the upper chest are the big pectoral muscles. Instead of being short and round as they are in undeveloped men, they would be broad and flat, extending from the breast bone to the armpit. If Grimek would raise his arm, the breast muscles could be seen to be joined, to almost flow into the shoulder muscles. Let us walk around him for a moment. What a back! The simple movement of raising and lowering the arms would show you a group of muscles which are far more than you thought possible. They would twist and turn and writhe about, but each one would be interconnected with the others. From the circle of the muscles of the upper back would extend the two "broadest of the back muscles," the latissimus group, which imparts the breadth and shapeliness to the upper back. The slope of the shoulders, the sweeping curve of the latissimus, is the mark of the really well- developed strength athlete. Square shoulders, hatrack in type, a perpendicular body, or even one slightly wedge-shaped, if broad shoulders are a natural part of the otherwise undeveloped frame instead of the swelling, sweeping curves of the Grimek back, are physical characteristics of the undeveloped man. The movement of these muscles shows them appearing in ever-changing contours. It is evident that they are well connected and interrelated.

The mid-section is much smaller, of course, than the upper back, but it is not small because it is lacking in muscles. It is so easy to see the powerful external oblique muscles, particularly strong in the case of Grimek, because he possesses the ability to thrust 300 pounds to one arm's length while bending to the side in the bent press position. Above these are the serratus magnus muscles, muscles which are invisible on the majority of humans. They connect with the ribs, and may seem to be ribs, but they are muscles and clearly defined in the Grimek physique. We pass below the waist and see a firm, well-rounded pair of gluteus maximus muscles. These, with the deep-lying muscles at the base of the spine—the spinae erecta—are the mark of a strong man.

Grimek has a most remarkable pair of legs. The calves are amazing, the thighs are almost as startling. It is difficult for you to tell where the thighs end and the hips begin. The muscles arise in one great sweeping curve from a position above the knee and extend well up into the hips. On the inside of the leg there is the superdevelopment of the sartorius muscles. On the back of the man there is a chain of powerful well-developed muscle from the ankle to the base of the neck, with all the muscles merging into one another. Every part of the body is adequately covered with muscles, muscles designed to move the body and limbs powerfully in many diverse manners. The muscles are symmetrical and, because of this symmetry, they are balanced and strong. Every muscle is strong, and because they are strong and well-developed, the entire effect is symmetrical. Symmetry and strength are closely allied. An all-around training program, designed to make one stronger or better built, will produce the combined effect about which I am writing.

CHAPTER NINE
Strength and Development As a Result of Natural Advantages

Some men gain very rapidly in strength and development. Their bodies are ready for exercise; through mode of living or heredity they have splendid internal processes. They gain immediately when they take up the practice of physical training. Adjustments must take place in the bodies of other individuals before they begin to make progress. I have been endeavoring to offer reasons for the great progress and lack of progress of various individuals. The condition of the mind, eating habits, inherited qualities are all reasons for the greater success of some as compared to others.

While it is true that any man can become strong even though he may be handicapped when he starts by being ill, narrow-shouldered, overweight, short or slender, those who are in the best condition in the beginning will gain most and with greatest rapidity. With proper living, including vigorous, progressive exercise, those who are sick will overcome their conditions and will become strong. Any healthy man can build muscle upon his body but some will gain more quickly than others.

Favorably endowed men such as Joe Miller who enlarged his chest a full twelve inches in a single year's time, Dave Mayor who gained quickly from 120 to 265, Terpak who was world's champion two years after he started serious weight training, Davis, who was world's champion before he was even United States champion, and of course Stanko who gained so sensationally, had natural advantages to begin with. Seldom do these men with natural advantages seriously take up the practice of physical training. They are too prone to be satisfied with the state of health that heredity or their mode of life has brought to them. Should these men with natural advantages become sufficiently interested they would quickly forge ahead to the top flight of the strength and development world.

Just what do I mean by natural advantages? First would be strong internal works, sound heart, good lungs, proper operation of all organs, good digestion and elimination, proper skeletal proportions, good size and inherited possibilities of splendid development.

Broad shoulders, after the internal efficiency concerning which I have written so much, are certainly distinct advantages. They are usually an indication of a large and sturdy bony framework, and a good chest on which there is plenty of room to build muscle. There usually is and always should be a close relation between the shoulders and the chest. When the chest is enlarged the shoulders broaden; when the shoulders are broad there must be a good chest below them. If you had very narrow shoulders it would not be natural for you to have a big chest, although you could have a deep chest. Early in life I was narrow-shouldered, so narrow that I was ridiculed by my playmates. I had a fair depth of chest ever since I can remember, the result of athletics during the growing years, but this chest was narrow and what is usually called chicken-breasted. Under those circumstances it is difficult to build a well-proportioned physique. How well I succeeded with hard and persistent effort is best proven by my present physique.

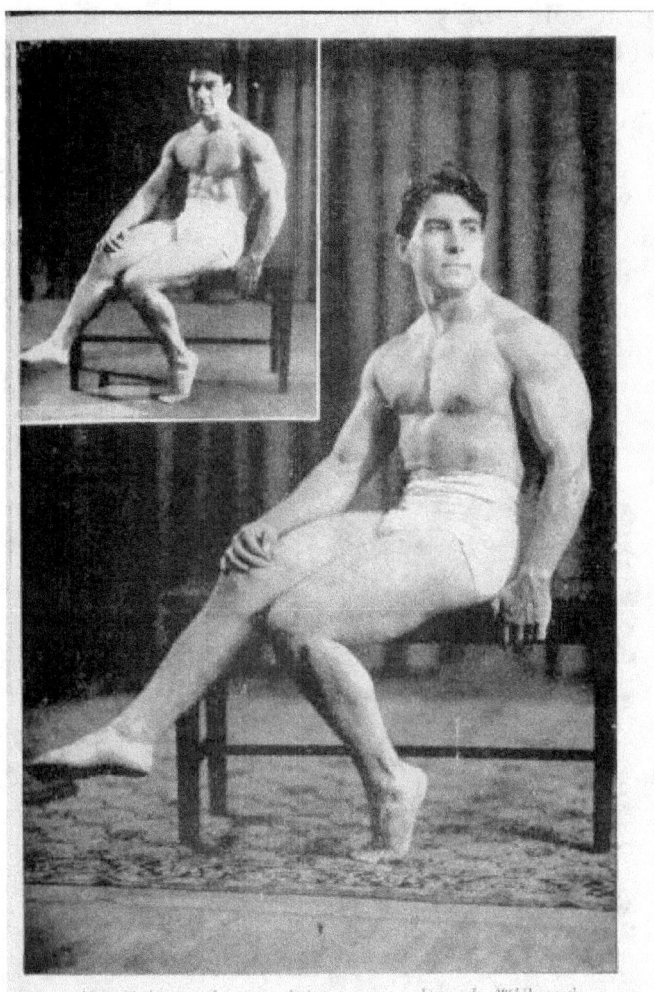

Tony Terlazzo as he appeared six years ago, and recently. While vastly stronger when the second photo was taken, 11 pounds heavier, only careful scrutiny of the photo will detect the fact that six years have passed with great physical improvement between the two.

All strong men are broad-shouldered and big-chested—most of all big-chested—but as I have said when men are big-chested they must be big-shouldered too. If you have broad shoulders when you start with progressive training as I teach it you already have several advantages: strength and vigor in the lungs of your big chest, more room for the organs in the mid-section of the body, more area on which to place muscles and the greater muscular leverage which comes from the spread of a good pair of shoulders. You have the advantage of possessing a good-looking physique to begin with, for any man with broad shoulders is potentially strong, has great possibilities of strength and can acquire this great strength if he will persist and develop all the muscles of the shoulders. I am referring chiefly to width of shoulder bones, rather than to apparently broad shoulders consisting of unusual depth to the deltoid or shoulder muscles.

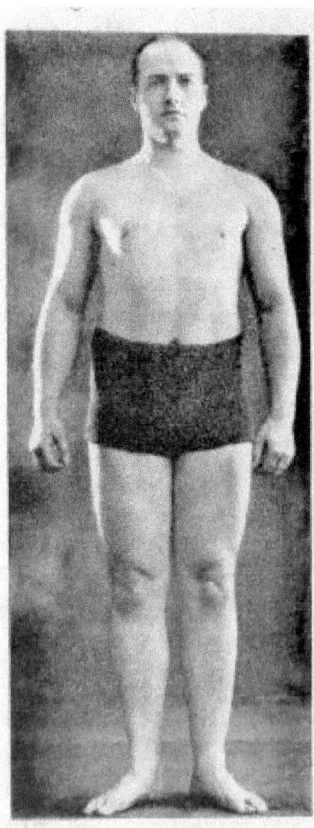

The author at 35 years of age at the start of his world-famous 20 weeks of training during which he established a world's record for physical gains as measured by strength, development, and lifting ability. In this photo he weighed 230, trained down to 225 in the first several weeks, and then built up to 243½ pounds as shown in the photo on the opposite page.

If you don't have broad shoulders you can obtain them through training. Even up to the age of fifty when there is of course no possibility of additional growth of the bones, adjustments take place in the shoulder assembly, the cartilages and attachments are lengthened and toughened so that definitely broader shoulders will result. Weighing 180 pounds at the age of twenty-one, now weighing 260 to 265, I have gained more than twelve inches in chest measurement during that period. I am not sure of my shoulder circumference at the age of twenty-one, but judge it was slightly more than the forty-two inches I measured around the shoulders in 1916, before entering the army and taking part in the World War, when I weighed 167 pounds. But now I measure fifty-eight inches around the shoulders, a gain of sixteen inches, all of it being made since I reached my present height and most of it being acquired after the age of twenty-one when many believe that it is no longer possible to gain in chest measurements or shoulder breadth. When these adjustments take place in the bony framework of the shoulder assembly, there is a possibility of gaining two inches in breadth and at least five inches in shoulder circumference by thickening and deepening the muscles on the point of the shoulders. In all the really strong men, particularly the weight lifters, there is a surprising depth to the shoulder muscles. The undeveloped man has deltoids only a part of an inch in thickness, but in the strength athlete they vary from one to two inches in depth.

Leverage is a very definite natural advantage. At times you see a man who lifts startling poundages and does not seem to have strength enough to do this. My pupil, Jack "Human Guinea Pig" Cooper, a young man of six feet four and a half inches in height, eighteen years of age, who weighed 155 at the beginning of his training, is the subject of a training demonstration. At first glance he would seem to have been the worst possible subject, but Jack did have

163

possibilities, a good pair of shoulders, very long legs and a comparatively short back—the type who would gain in strength quickly but find it difficult to acquire the weight his frame should include.

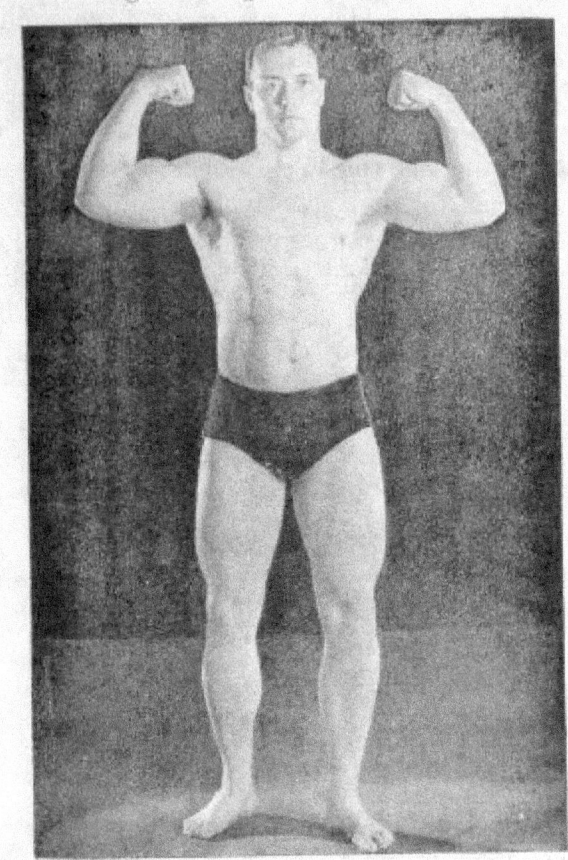

Bob Hoffman, just after his 36th birthday and at the completion of his 20 weeks of intensive weight training. He followed the York courses exactly as they have been offered to hundreds of thousands of York pupils.

My expectations have been realized, for Jack has succeeded with some wonderful lifts. In a year's training time his lifts gained to 230 press, 260 snatch and 330 clean and jerk. A splendid and truly amazing lifting total, particularly when elevated by one so youthful and in such a limited period of

164

training—a lifting total of 820. Few are the men in this nation, or the world for that matter, who lift as much. Jack's gain of fifty-two pounds during this period, a pound a week, is most pleasing, but now his gains will be slower and more difficult to attain. He has improved greatly with this additional weight of fifty-two pounds upon his elongated frame, but could easily use another fifty pounds and still be on the lean side. When I look at Jack in the gymnasium I have said, "Jack, you have truly become amazing. One would think that you were pretty good if you pressed 175, snatched 200 and clean and jerked 260. But 230, 260, 330; that hardly seems possible." Jack does not look powerful enough to lift the weights he handles. He has a combination of physical attributes which have helped him reach the heights—physical advantages of broad shoulders, short back and long legs. The short back permits good leverage; the long legs let him pull the weight high and at the same time he can dip low under it. Both in the snatch and the clean this is an advantage. The longer-legged fellows with shorter backs can usually pull the weights best. But added to this are Jack's broad shoulders and his long but properly balanced arms. So he is able to do well on the press and well enough on the jerk that this should keep pace with his cleaning ability. I should say that Jack Cooper has natural advantages, but without hard and intelligent, persistent training he would have naturally gained five or ten pounds and still be tall, skinny and frail.

With fair width of bones in the shoulders to start with, proper exercise consisting of bar bells, dumbells and cables, with the many diverse movements this equipment offers, powerful muscles will be developed on the point of the shoulders, but the bony framework too will become much wider. Our discussion up to this point has taken into consideration only men of maturity. When the young fellows who are still in the growing stage take up the practice of weight training, their growth is sure to be greatly stimulated. This rapid growth invariably takes place in the bodies of young men at the growing stage, and younger brothers who are inspired by their elders to start weight training always grow considerably larger and stronger than their father and older brothers.

When a man has built thick, well-developed, powerful deltoids, he is certain to have a good rib box, for so many of the exercises which develop the deltoids are good breathing exercises which rapidly increase the size of the chest. There is a close connection between deltoid movements and those of the chest and upper back, for all of these muscles have common attachments. In starting out to develop the deltoids, thus widening the shoulders, you are sure to develop the rib box and all the muscles that cover it, both on the chest and the back. And with broader shoulders and a bigger, deeper chest you become bigger all over. Therefore it is evident that a man who has good shoulders and a big, round, deep chest to begin with, has natural advantages which will permit him to forge ahead in his training as compared to another who does not have these natural advantages.

The deltoids' chief function is to raise the arms to the front or side or overhead. They receive some benefit in slowly lowering weights, but they do not pull the arms down. The large muscles of the back, known as the latissimus dorsi, perform this function. Therefore the cable exercise in which the arms held straight are pulled from overhead to shoulder height is the best developer of this particular muscle group which imparts such a breadth and pleasing curve to the upper back.

While most persons measure a man's strength by the breadth of his shoulders, few realize that broad hips are

166

also essential to strength. Most persons, novelists in particular, seem to feel that a man's body should be wedge-shaped, tapering from broad, sloping shoulders to a very narrow waist and with narrow hips. A man who has narrow hips to begin with can develop power by developing the buttock muscles, scientifically termed the gluteus maximus. These muscles while remaining narrow will become very deep.

But if the hip bones themselves are big, the man has natural advantages which aid him to become strong. They also help him become fat too if he does nothing about conditioning his body. Heavy hip bones and a broad pelvis which forms a foundation for the organs of the abdominal region, placing the legs wide apart, permit the legs to carry much more muscle than if the pelvis is narrow and the bones close together. The width of the pelvis affects a man's strength, for it gives him a much firmer foundation, and he stands much more solidly. You can easily understand this for it is much easier to upset a high narrow table than one of the same height which is broader, just as it is easier to upset a narrow-hipped man than a broad-hipped one.

A man with upper thigh bones which extend out a bit from knee to hips is stronger than a man with vertical bones. A woman's bones flare out to the side much more than a man's, to provide additional room in the abdominal cavity, which is why so many women have heavy thigh muscles. This is the chief place where women are strong and you will frequently find young women who can out- push men of their age and greater weight. I have seen girls who were members of a gymnastic team push much heavier men all around the gym and the male gymnast who fancied he was strong was powerless to prevent them. Similarly I have seen Gracie Bard, the Strength and Health model, who is rather a small girl, only five feet two, 114 pounds in weight, yet is the possessor of powerful lower limbs, chiefly as a result of professional dancing, but also due to the fact that she always enjoyed physical exercise and sports, and spent considerable time at weight training, have no difficulty in even upsetting some of the young boxers of our boxing team, who thought that with their masculine strength they should be able to resist her efforts very successfully. But they were far from as strong as they should have been.

Young men who are destined to be fat if they do nothing about their natural advantages frequently have hips which are quite a bit larger than their chests. Physical training would enlarge their chests and shoulders and such men could possess most attractive physiques. There should not be more than two or three inches' difference in the hip measurement and the chest when the tape is passed around the body just below the armpits. Our really strong men of the past and present had big square hips. Arthur Saxon and George Hackenschmidt in the past and Dave Mayor and Steve Stanko of the present are men who had the advantages of big hips to begin with. While there was a difference of just five inches in the hip and chest measurement of Sandow—forty-four-inch chest and thirty-nine-inch hips —Hackenschmidt who had big hips also had a phenomenally large chest with probably ten inches' difference between the measurements of these two parts of his body. Oscar Mathes, another great old timer, who has a just claim to the title, "Father of American Weight Lifting," was very short and quite powerful, only five feet in height, and had a forty-inch chest and thirty-five-inch hips. I number Mr. Mathes among my very best friends at present. He is seventy-seven years of age, has been married fifty-five years, and is superhealthy, strong, active and an enthusiast concerning strength at present as during all of his long life. He is a real link between the present and the glamorous strength days of the past.

Big hands are an advantage in the acquisition of strength if they are also accompanied by long fingers. Big hands can more easily be developed into powerful parts but the fact that you might have small hands or short fingers is no bar to strength. John Davis, the world's light-heavyweight and United States champion, has rather short fingers. Bob Mitchell, a member of the Olympic team of 1936, senior national champion of 1934 and a record holder at quick lifts, had small, almost girlish hands. Warren Lincoln Travis has short-fingered hands but he has developed them to the point where he excels at many forms of strength tests in which gripping power and finger strength are involved. Frank Kay, runner-up in the junior and senior national 181-pound weight lifting championships, one of the world's best lifters, has amazingly small hands and short fingers. Some men have hands which are strong in one way, yet weak in another. John Marx, great old time strong man, had hands of enormous power with long fingers, so that he excelled at lifting thick-handled dumbells. A dumbell with a three-inch handle he possessed was beyond the efforts of all other strong men to lift. He was also credited with breaking coins and horseshoes. Yet Cyclops Bienski, another strong man of the same period, had short fingers while also excelling at chain and coin breaking.

Of our present men of strength, none has a stronger grip than John Grimek. It is reasonable to believe that much of this gripping power is the result of his phenomenal forearm development, for as explained in another chapter the attachments of the finger muscles are in the forearm. My own grip was never particularly strong before taking up the practice of weight lifting. In spite of having excelled at rowing, which should have developed a good grip, I could not hang by the grip of one hand. I remember a short time after I started with bar bells I could only one hand dead lift

140 pounds, for my weak grip restricted my lifting, while a young friend and my business partner who had been a plumber most of his life and had a great grip could lift the entire 225-pound weight of the bar bell. Yet a year later I discovered on a visit to Coney Island and Warren Lincoln Travis that I could lift weights in some of his gripping tests that others of my group could not elevate.

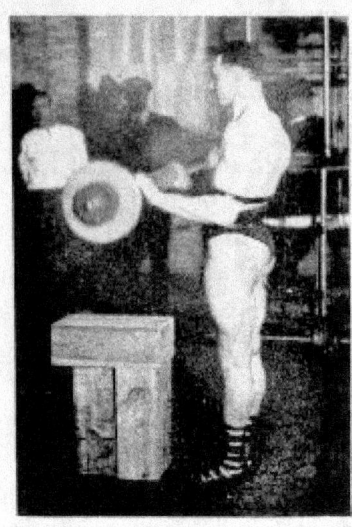

Antone Matysek, who had one of the most famous physiques of all time, setting a record as a strength show in 1926, in the back hand curl, with elbows bound to the sides. He is now a police officer in Baltimore, Md.

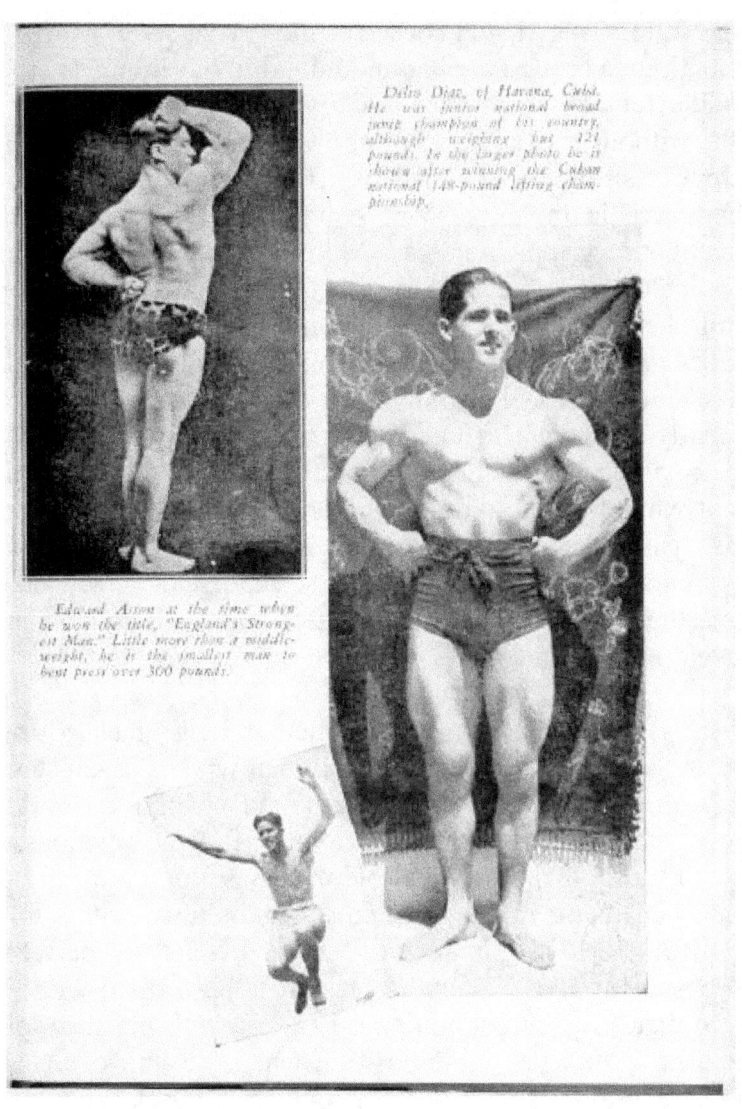

Delio Diaz, of Havana, Cuba. He was junior national broad jump champion of his country, although weighing but 121 pounds. In the larger photo he is shown after winning the Cuban national 148-pound lifting championship.

Edward Aston at the time when he won the title, "England's Strongest Man." Little more than a middleweight, he is the smallest man to bent press over 300 pounds.

During most of my lifting career I have lifted with what is known as the hook grip, wrapping the thumb around the bar, and then the fingers around the thumb. I can clean and jerk twenty more pounds with the hook than without it and snatch fifteen pounds more with the hook than without it.

Most lifters use what is known as the get set style, wrapping their fingers around the bar and hooking, but Johnny Terpak, middleweight king for the last five years, makes his great lifts without the hook grip, showing that he has unusual gripping strength. But this does not seem to be a natural characteristic in his case; it seems that he developed his exceptional gripping power. More than likely working in the coal mines in his early life during summer vacations while he was going to school and for some time afterward helped build this unusual grip. I have found that I do not have an exceptional grip in lifting thin-shafted bar bells, but recently on a visit to Ottawa, Canada, I was able to lift a thick-handled bar bell weighing 202 pounds a foot from the floor when I was told that no other man had been able to do this. It is evident that big strong hands if possessed in the beginning are a great adjunct to strength, but if you don't have them you can make the best of what you do have and develop an unusual grip.

There is a big question about whether long or short arms are an advantage. There are strong men who have unusually long arms. John Terry, the 132-pound champion, world's record holder in the two hands dead lift at 600 pounds, is one of these. It is quite possible that these long arms are an important factor in his great power and ability in this form of lifting. He is small of course to be so perfectly proportioned at 132 pounds. The lift is performed with the large plates of the international bar, and with his very long arms he is in a favorable position when the start of the lift is made. Of course he is very strong in the back too, for he can perform repetition dead lifts in the stiff-legged style with 500 pounds—good proof that he has unusual power in his back.

I believe that these long arms are a handicap in pressing, for his official best press of 190, while good, is twenty-five pounds back of the American record, also the world's best on record, of 215 pounds established by Tony Terlazzo way back in 1936 when he lifted as a featherweight. But the long arms apparently are not a handicap in snatching and cleaning, for Terry established a world's two hands snatch record of 215 pounds in the world's championship at Vienna, and has pulled to the shoulder more than the world's record in the clean and jerk. Jack Cooper has long arms, but has the proper proportions of shoulder width and arm bones, and the long arms seem to be an advantage rather than a hindrance. Ronald Walker of England, former world's record holder in the two hands snatch, was built very much like Jack Cooper.

Very short arms can be a handicap. Gregory George is a great presser, having made his start this year in the national championships with the great poundage of 270. He has succeeded with 290 in good style and made 300 with a back bend. Yet this very shortness of arms which makes it possible for him to press so well is a handicap in cleaning (pulling the weight to the chest in one movement). His arms are so huge and so short that he cannot hold the bar upon his chest and when a weight of well over 300 pounds is reached he often misses his clean. At times he has made three misses and he lost this year's junior national title which he seemed to have "in the bag" because he could not hold the weight upon his shoulders. Men with very short arms are good pressers but they are all lacking in pulling power. Of the very short men, Firpo Lemma, national 112-pound champion for the last two years, has pressed 210 which is a world's record by a big margin, but he can never clean more than perhaps five pounds in excess of this amount, and his two hands snatch is only 140.

It is evident for all-around proficiency that you will have natural advantages if your arms are the proper length in relation to your height. Proper length is usually considered to be when the distance from outstretched finger tip to outstretched finger tip of the other hand when the hands are held level with the shoulder is the same as that of one's height. Years ago my reach was exactly the same as my height. Considering my narrower than normal shoulders at that time for my height, and the shortness of the upper arm bone, it is evident that I had longer than normal arms, particularly very long forearms. I have just measured for the first time in many years and find that my reach is three inches greater than my height—the result of a considerable gain in shoulder breadth. Now my leverage is a bit more favorable which accounts for part of the fact that my two arm pressing ability, formerly the world's worst, has crept up to 200 pounds, with a bit of back bend.

I have discussed briefly the fact that long legs combined with a short back produce favorable leverage, yet Jack Cooper's long legs are not as favorable or as well balanced as mine, it would seem. We are the same height at the knee. Jack is a full inch taller than I, yet he is 2.5 inches longer from the knee to hip than I. With the same length of lower leg bone, 2.5 inches longer upper leg bone, his back of course is 1.5 inches shorter than mine, probably more than this as Jack has a longer neck.

The leaders in weight lifting are of many shapes, sizes, types and designs. Each has learned to make the most of his natural advantages and to overcome to the best of his ability his disadvantages. That's why some men use the split style, some the squat; others press with a close grip, some with a wide grip; some jerk the weight from the chest, others from the shoulders. Each man must try the various methods of lifting or of other athletics and adopt a style which permits him to make the greatest showing.

174

CHAPTER TEN
Strength Through Quality of Muscle

Why is one man of a given body weight and identical muscular measurements so much stronger than another man? Tony Terlazzo is Olympic, world's, North American and United States weight lifting champion. He holds the world's record in the two hands press-at 255 pounds in the 148-pound class. A large percentage of the male population of the world is of this weight which might be termed the average weight. Yet Tony has pressed officially seventeen pounds more weight than any other man of his weight in the world's history. He has elevated 340 pounds to arm's length overhead—forty-five pounds more than double his body weight.

Jack "Human Guinea Pig" Cooper, six feet four and a half inches in height, eighteen years of age, weight at the time of writing this chapter 207, has gained fifty-two pounds in a little more than a year. He is the subject at present of a training experiment or demonstration which has already met with great success. A member of our team, he has made lifts of 230 press, 260 two hands snatch and 330 clean and jerk. But he is far from satisfied. He weighs more than the 196 pounds life insurance charts list as the correct weight for a man of his height. His lifts are truly extraordinary but he craves most of all increased body weight and greater muscular size. His greatest lament is the fact that his flexed arm measures only a little over fourteen inches. He desires arms which compare more favorably with the eighteen-inch arms of Grimek and Stanko or the nineteen-inch arms of Dave Mayor. Yet he has acquired one phase of strength which has created continued amazement among those who see him in action.

When the uninitiated hear of the great poundages the champions lift, their usual remark is, "There's a lot of knack to lifting weights, isn't there?" And my invariable reply is, "There's some knack, but strength is most important." A man who is strong and has no form or knack can lift more than a man with less strength and superlative form. Although I have had a most successful athletic career, reaching the heights in a number of well-known branches of sport, my weight lifting career from its earliest inception has proven that I was not strong, but won rather through skill, form or knack, unusual endurance and rapid recuperative powers which were the result of proper training and right living. After having won national championships in a number of sports, having been a boxing champion, I could not properly press eighty pounds with two hands, and after a year of training, 115 was my two hands press record. Most men can do better at the very beginning or after a few weeks of training.

Now my best records are 200 press, 230 snatch, 300 clean and jerk. Those who have seen me in action admit that I have splendid form; never did a big man move faster or assume lower lifting positions; with a lifetime of athletic experience I possess the ability to greatly outdo myself when it is necessary, but with all the attributes of a champion, except great strength, my lifts are far behind the best records of the leading heavyweights. Steve Stanko has pressed 300, snatched 305, clean and jerked 375. The latter two are world's records. What does he possess that I do not have? He weighs thirty pounds less, he isn't quite as tall, his arm is slightly larger, his chest and thighs a bit smaller, but he constantly lifts world's record poundages.

Quality of muscle is the chief reason why one lifter or one athlete excels another. Jack Cooper from his appearance and muscular size would be considered a very good lifter if he hoisted 200 snatch and 260 clean and jerk, yet his records are 260 in the former and 330 in the latter. He has favorable leverage, it is admitted, long legs and a short back, which help his pull, he has broad shoulders and proper balance in length of his arm bones which will make him in time a great presser and contender for the world's championship, but it would never be expected that he possessed the great strength which permits him to elevate such tremendous weights overhead.

There are other strength stars who surprise the spectators when they are in action. Johnny Terpak, who won the world's middleweight championship in Paris, and has been United States champion during the years of 1936-37-38-39 and 40, weighs as little as 152 when lifting in that class. He's nicely formed but certainly does not look strong enough to two hands snatch 260 and clean and jerk 330. John Terry for the last three years has been the United States 132-pound champion. In Vienna he established a world's record of 215 pounds in the two hands snatch. He has definitely proven that he is the strongest man in the world of his weight. And his greatest claim to fame is his world's record of 600 pounds in the two hands dead weight lift, a weight which is scores of pounds heavier than any other man in the world of his weight has been able to lift.

John Davis, who won the world's 181-pound lifting title at Vienna, in the Middle Atlantic championships last year cleaned (pulled to the shoulder in one movement, considered to be the hardest part of the lift) a weight of 370 pounds. This was more than double his body weight and he is the largest lifter in the world who has pulled more than double his body weight to his chest in this style. In fact, at that time, only two other men in the world had pulled such a great weight to their chests in the same style: Charles Rigoulot, the French professional champion, who, using a

177

springy bar ten feet long, had lifted a greater weight, and Steve Stanko who since has established world's records of 371 and 375 in the clean and jerk.

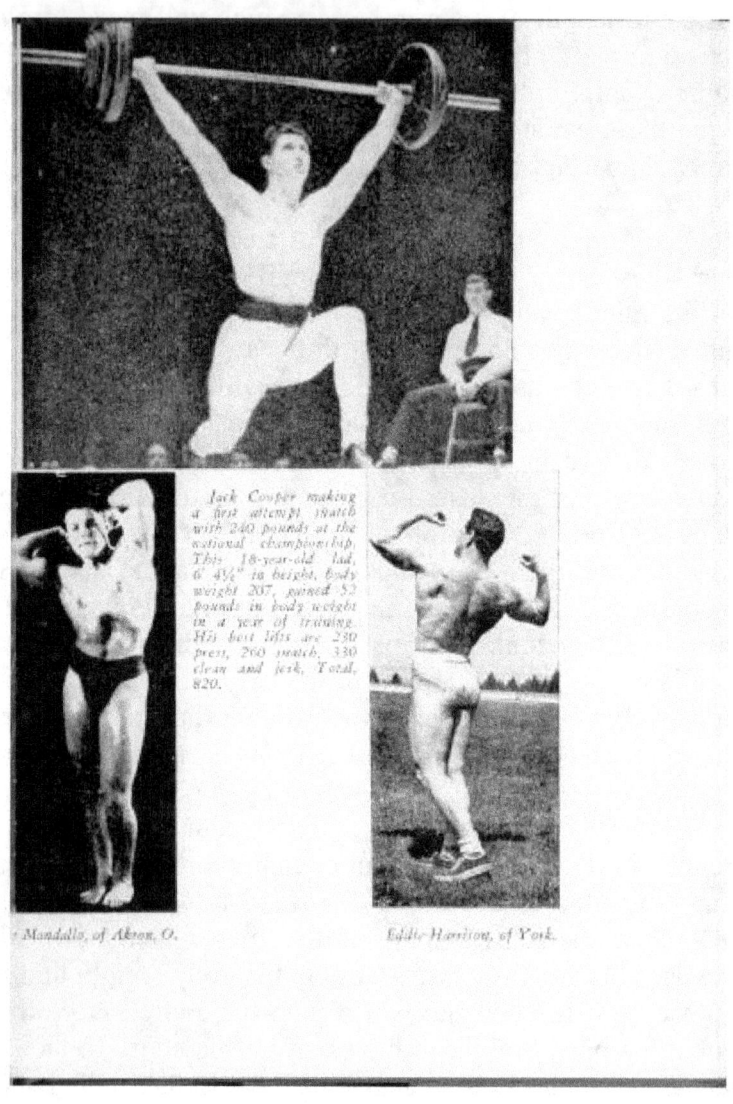

Jack Cooper making a first attempt snatch with 240 pounds at the national championship. This 18-year-old lad, 6' 4½" in height, body weight 207, gained 52 pounds in body weight in a year of training. His best lifts are 230 press, 260 snatch, 330 clean and jerk, Total, 820.

Mandalla, of Akron, O.   Eddie Harrison, of York.

Roy Hall of our Canadian team, the Toronto-York lifting team, was another of these mysterious lifters who did not appear strong enough to elevate the poundages he habitually put overhead. Weighing a bit over 170 he one arm clean and jerked 215 pounds and two arm snatched 250 pounds—remarkable feats of strength for a tall man of such slender frame, with only a fourteen-and-a-half-inch arm. Another of the world's great lifters, Hans Haas of Austria, who in 1928 was the first man in the world to clean and jerk double body weight, lifting 297 at the Olympic Games while competing in the 148-pound class, was another amazing lifter. He at one time had six of the seven world's records in the 148-pound class, and the one hand clean and jerk record in the next heavier class, the 165. He was the greatest one hand lifter of all time. He holds the world's one hand clean and jerk record at 237 pounds, 148-pound class, exactly the same poundage as the world's record in the 181-pound class, and, weighing just over the 148-pound limit, he lifted 248 pounds in the one hand lift. This great poundage is 3.5 pounds less than the one hand clean and jerk record in the heavyweight class, which of course means that this comparatively small lifter, tall for his weight, made the second best lift in all recorded weight lifting history in this style of lifting, being exceeded only by a man who outweighed him by a hundred pounds.

Joe Mills, the great Central Falls, Rhode Island, lifter, has only a thirteen-inch upper arm yet has pressed 205 with two hands and clean and jerked 265, double his body weight. Ralph Scull of St. Hedwig's Y.M.C.A., Elizabeth, New Jersey, the junior national champion of 1940, runner up in the seniors the same year, has two hands snatched 205, clean and jerked 265, and is tall and slender for his weight. Bob Knodle, who was senior national champion in the 112- and 118-pound class years ago, was another of these mystery lifters. Tall, slender, with little apparent de-

179

velopment, he won titles and established records year after year.

In England there have been some little men who lifted almost unbelievable poundages. J. H. Holliday of Manchester, England, with only a thirteen-and-a-half-inch arm, bent pressed 203 pounds. W. L. Carquest with an arm only a quarter inch larger was successful with 196 pounds. W. L. Pullum, at a body weight of 126, elevated 225 in the bent press style.

In any class of men we are considering, who possessed quality of muscle, we cannot leave out Arthur Saxon, the great bent presser, who at a body weight of 210, quite small as compared to the 300 pounds of Louis Cyr and Louis Uni, established a world's professional record of 371 in the bent press; or John Y. Smith, the great old timer from Boston.

These men all had something that other men did not have—not just weight, for they competed against and defeated men who outweighed them by many pounds. Quality of muscle was the answer. It is natural that you should wonder the why and the wherefore, the how, of this quality of muscle possessed by the champions and the leading strength stars of the day. Why am I not as strong as Steve Stanko, why does Tony Terlazzo excel the world? Part of the reason why I don't lift more in proportion to a man like Stanko is the fact that I learned of weight lifting comparatively late in life, at a time when I was engaged in a business which required a great deal of travelling. Now my work is travelling, writing, lecturing, teaching, my time is taken up, so that frequently I miss weeks of training. It is remarkable that I lift as much as I do under the circum- stances, but with the same training as Steve I would not be able to lift as well. Only one man can be champion; he's the champion of the world, and hard, heavy, persistent training has given him the power, the quality of muscle, to surpass the world in his favorite sport.

Without this explanation many men will wonder why they are not as strong as their friends who are of the same weight and have apparently the same muscular development. At all stages of life there are men who excel all those with whom they come in contact because they have this quality of muscle. At times the difference in apparent strength comes about because one man does not know how to apply his strength, while the other man has the gift of co-ordination, judgment of distance and timing which permits him to outperform the other fellow. This ability, in my own case, has permitted me to win from stronger men so many times, but a stronger man with the same ability and skill would easily have beaten me. Like the case of a good big man being better than a good little man, a man with quality of muscle will always outscore the man with less muscular strength providing he possesses a fair amount of skill or knack at his particular sport.

Muscles of the same size can be of high, intermediate or low quality. Just as there is a difference in a steel spring, an elastic cable, a musical instrument, or the famous sword blades of old as compared to an ordinary sword, muscles vary in strength. Sixty-five per cent of the men who make their beginning with progressive weight training seek to increase their body weight. Years ago, and in some quarters at present I am sorry to say, increased body weight is the fetish which is sought by the devotees of this type of training—increased weight at any price; live a life not too unlike that of a big pig; eat large quantities of food many times a day; be as lethargic as possible at all other times; drink, eat and sleep much, be slow moving, and perform a few heavy exercises three times a week. It was the published belief of the men who promoted this system of training that when once the increased body weight was obtained, the fat could be changed to muscle and the man's figure and proportions improved. But fat is a different substance from muscle; it cannot be changed into muscle. Rather long and painful effort is required to wear the fat away and replace it with the muscle which should have been developed in the first place. The company who advocated this system of training was able to sell more weights and larger sets of weights, with increased profits to themselves, which was their chief object.

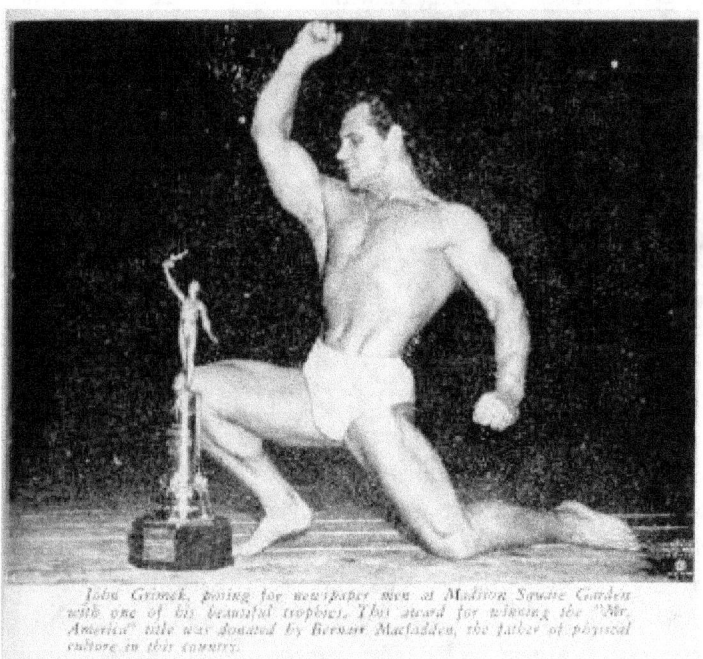

John Grimek, posing for newspaper men at Madison Square Garden with one of his beautiful trophies. This award for winning the "Mr. America" title was donated by Bernarr Macfadden, the father of physical culture in this country.

There are other physical directors who offer courses of training without apparatus, consisting of high repetitions in all the exercises. It is much more profitable to sell a few printed pages for prices ranging from twenty-five dollars if you act quickly down to five dollars or even less if you wait a while, than it is to sell heavy, "expensive to build, pack

182

and ship" weights. It was discovered years ago that, while a two- or even a five-pound dumbell would only provide enough resistance to build the muscles to sufficient size and strength to perform exercises with that weight, muscle could be built faster if at the completion of each movement extreme contraction of the muscle would be made. Then it was discovered that similar results could be had without apparatus. Larger-sized muscles could be obtained this way than with free-hand movements alone. The use of the will in vigorously tensing the muscles at the end of each movement, making them work harder, added somewhat to the size of the muscle. But it did not develop all the muscles and the body of the athlete who followed such a system benefited just a little, usually in the earlier days of the training program, but did not have strength which was commensurate with the apparent development.

I have received a host of letters from such individuals who were surprised to learn that another man with the same size arm or measurements even smaller than they could elevate so much more weight overhead. The latter man had a more balanced development, greater strength in the muscles, tendons and ligaments. The first man had only coarse, inflated tissue.

The "train you by mail" business has run its course for years with most systems being designed only to increase the body weight or even the size of the most apparent muscles, which never results in the gaining of maximum strength and development. The courses of exercise designed to increase the strength of the muscles, but providing little in the way of increased size and shapeliness, have passed along. For the majority of men and women do exercise to build their bodies, and hard work which does not bring the desired increases in size and shapeliness is decidedly unpopular. A few systems which inflate the tissue, while adding little to the strength and offering very little in the way of shapeliness, still flourish, but they are losing in popularity with each passing year. The third and the ideal way is the one that I and all who tried the other methods prefer. This is a system of training which not only brings a muscle to its greatest size and its best proportions, but also produces enormous strength.

It is estimated that all humans, large or small, old or young, developed or undeveloped, possess the same number of muscular fibres—four billion. If you don't believe me, count them for yourself. The difference in body weight or strength comes about through the improvement in size and strength of these billions of muscular fibres. The thickness of the individual fibres which compose the muscle determines its size. It is much easier to increase the size of these fibres than their strength. Many men have gained rapidly in the first year in size until to the uninitiated they look as strong as the muscles of a real strong man. But there is a difference. I am offering two photos of Tony Terlazzo which illustrate this point. The first photo was taken in 1934 and shows Tony at a body weight of 137 at the time when he became the third man in the history of the world to clean and jerk double body weight, succeeding that year with 275 pounds. His press record then was 215 and snatch record 212. Unless you examine both photos very carefully, the one taken this year (1940) —six years later—is little different. The six years have made little change in his face; he looks alive and alert, his face un- marked and unlined in spite of six years of world's championship lifting performances. In the second photo Tony weighs 148, a gain of eleven pounds. It is so well distributed that its location is hard to notice. But his lifting records, made in official competition, have soared to 255 press, 250 snatch, 340 clean and jerk—a total of 845 as compared to 695 six years ago. The added pounds so well distributed over his body, and the improved quality of muscle, have made this great gain in weight lifting ability.

Gains are made very rapidly in the beginning of physical training. There are countless examples of men who have gained from six to twelve inches in chest circumference in a single year's training, and with such a gain in chest development the shoulders broaden and the limbs become much larger, with a great increase in strength. Some weight may be added with additional years of training, but the usual result is an improved moulding of the muscles, an added shapeliness, better quality muscles, an increase in strength, a growth in the measurement of the flexed muscle, with less gain in body weight.

The majority of young men who have used their muscles but little will gain an average of a pound a week in three months of training—thirteen pounds in all—if they follow the system of training all York Bar Bell men are urged to practice. Starting with a moderate weight, just the amount the untrained muscles can easily handle for five repetitions, with alternate training days and days of rest, the poundages and the counts are increased progressively, gradually giving them longer and harder periods of training, and the muscles grow in strength and size.

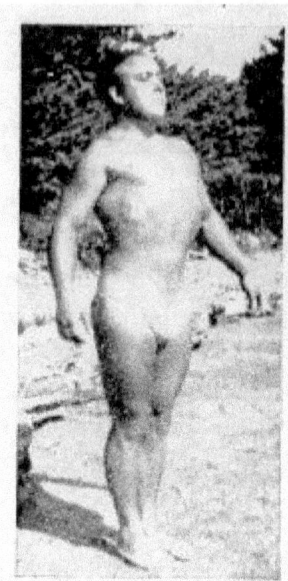

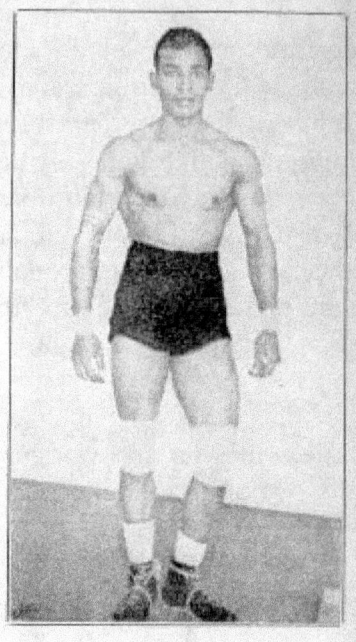

Shamr, the great Egyptian weight lifter. Weighing 143, he cleaned 340 pounds. Only his comparatively poor pressing and jerking ability prevented him from beating the great York lifter, Tony Terlazzo, in the world's championships.

Tommy Pedder of Bellville, Ont., Canada, a long distance swimmer who trains with barbells. He was United States junior national weight lifting champion.

Tommy is only 5 feet tall yet has built himself into a miniature Sandow.

The only proper way to develop the body is with a system of training such as I have briefly described, some method which permits graduated increases in resistance, with rest periods in between during which the worn and broken down tissue is replaced. Too many men have wasted their time on methods designed only to pump up the muscles a bit, but not to really develop the strength or the quality of the muscle with the improved shapeliness that is sure to result. While most of these muscle tensing exercises have disappeared they have been practiced by so many millions of men that they deserve at least a passing comment here. The first regular exercise I followed was called the Swoboda system. This Swoboda should not be confused

186

with the great Viennese weight lifter by that name, a man who weighed 400 pounds and jerked over 400 pounds. This Swoboda was a man who merely adopted that name. His course consisted of tensing movements. You can try the method for a moment if you wish. Clench your fist, bend your arm, bring the fist close to the shoulder. With this movement you are bringing into action the flexor muscles of the arm which are called the biceps. After you have bent the arm to its fullest extent, harden the muscle so that it will, after a bit of practice, rise up into an elongated hump or bump. Continue this movement until the muscle is tired. By practicing this movement for a full month, exercising every day, you will gain the ability to hump the muscle up a bit more, and the tape will show a gain in measurement. This increase in size is particularly evident when the muscle is under tension but the muscle itself, after you have acquired the ability to flex it with ever greater force, will result in a somewhat larger tape measurement. Persistence with this movement will make it possible for you to show a very imposing bump.

The practice of these movements very early in life built for me what my brothers laughingly called "manufactured bumps." I had a bump on my arm, about as big as a walnut, of which I was very proud. My father spent years in following such exercises and did acquire the ability to contract his muscles in a startling way. He was very proud of his muscles, and showed them to all and sundry with or without an excuse. But I happen to know that he did not possess strength commensurate with his apparent development, and it is quite evident that I did not gain strength through years of persistent practice with tensing exercises. If I had only known what I know now, and what you know now if you read my books and follow the courses they contain, I would have saved much effort and accomplished so much more.

With the tensing system, similar movements were possible with all the voluntary muscles. It was necessary to learn something about muscle control in order to perform these movements properly. Men, who had developed their strength through the lifting of weights, offered tensing courses, claiming as one advertiser today does that he merely demonstrates his strength in his three times weekly training with weights. The powerful men who offered these courses had lifted weights, exercised with weights, used cable expanders, wrestled, tumbled, hand balanced and practiced a wide variety of body-building sports and exercises. Their advertising created great confusion; ambitious body builders did not know whom to believe. Progress was slow, but the years have proven to anyone who investigated a reasonable amount, that progressive resistance which really tries the strength of a muscle is the only sure way to obtain maximum results.

Muscles acquired by free-hand movements or tensing may seem large when measured with the tape, but when relaxed they are different. There is not the rounded, well-developed, powerful appearance to be seen in the muscle of the man who has developed himself with real exercise, weight lifting or progressive cable training or with other apparatus which lends itself well to graded resistance. The muscle which is developed through tensing stands up in a sharp bump, while the man who has real strength in his muscles, the result of hard work or proper exercise, has muscles of an entirely different shape and a great deal more strength: he has developed quality of muscle.

I have known men who had fifteen-inch arms developed through tensing exercises who did not have nearly as much strength as men with thirteen-inch arms who built their strength and development through weight training.

My chief interest is in the building of better bodies for the men who train with me. The desired results of physical training I would list as follows: Shapeliness, increased strength and added weight. I believe in an all-around training program which will first of all build a symmetrical physique, a physique which will be shapely every pound of the way as it progresses to greater strength and added body weight. I urge the men who follow my instruction to practice an all-around training system, to strive for all desirable physical qualities simultaneously. Such a system will quickly build a shapeliness to the body, quality of muscle and strength which will attract favorable attention wherever seen.

CHAPTER ELEVEN
All-Around Development

Those who have seen the advanced York bar bell man in action are always impressed with his great strength, athletic ability, fine appearance and extraordinary development. Every York man who has trained for any length of time has a physique which attracts favorable attention wherever it is seen. While most men and women prefer shapeliness first, as do I, there are many men who have been misled and have followed a system of training which will not bring out the limit in shapeliness and development. I am fascinated by strength, a lover of strength feats and a great admirer of the really strong man, but I prefer a man who is shapely with that strength.

Although all the members of the York team, who this year startled the world by winning all the United States titles, are my very intimate friends and close associates, I see more of Steve Stanko and John Grimek than any of the others. They are frequent visitors at my home. In these two close friends we have two of the best-built men in the world and two of the strongest. Steve Stanko certainly is the world's strongest lifter, and it is doubtful if there is a man anywhere in the world who excels him in sheer power. He has a magnificent physique, weighs 225 pounds at his height of approximately six feet, and maintains a slender waistline in spite of his great strength and splendid appetite. I have impressed it upon him, and been more than ably seconded by our mutual friend, John Grimek, that his shapeliness is even more important than his strength; that he must maintain his attractive physique and not permit himself to get overweight and out of shape as the continental European heavyweight lifters have done. Grimek, who recently won the most highly publicized and most representative contest to find the best-built man in America, at the national contest at Madison Square Garden, is a really strong man too, as best proven by his military press of 285 pounds. He was one of the place winners in the lifting contest. These two men have combined splendid proportions, bodies which are making them immortal, and great strength. Other York men who are leading lifters, the strongest men in the land, are also the best-built. Terlazzo who has proven his power many times in winning lifting titles was winner in his class at the best-built man championships at Chicago last year. He was among the leaders in similar contests. The men I have enumerated and many others—Bachtell, Levan, Terry, Davis, Venables, Zagurski, Farnham, Harrison, Terpak—prove that all-around training brings best results.

I have seen and you must have seen many individuals who while showing no pronounced muscular development are quite strong. I can partially admire such men, as I am a lover of strength, but at every opportunity I urge them to change their systems of living and training so that they will obtain all-around favorable results. Such men have performed work or exercise which has strengthened the tendons, ligaments and cartilages but has not provided enough movement of the muscles, enough tensing or working from the extreme of contraction to the extreme of extension to really develop the muscles. You have seen such men. Among any group of hard-working men will be found one or two, or three or four, depending upon the size of the group who are stronger than the others. If you have been present at tug of war contests where men from the factories and police departments were in action you have seen such men. Each year at the Canadian national exhibition at Toronto I witness the tug of war contests. Few of these men are well balanced in their development, but they are usually big-boned and heavy—thick-set but not the well-built athletic type of man we are accustomed to see in professional strong men, or our great amateur lifters. These men are strong and have the ability to move heavy loads, to lift, push or carry surprising weights. Their training has resulted in the development of powerful ligaments.

It was powerful ligaments and tendons which won the title, "Strongest Man in All of New England" for John Y. Smith, for three of the tests were the left hand dead lift, the right hand dead lift, and the two hands dead lift with knuckles front—all movements in which the poundage hoisted was limited by the gripping power. Smith had been a sailing ship man in the old days and had developed great strength in his muscular attachments, which has made it possible for him to gain and retain strength fame for a lifetime. After leaving the sea he was at one time a professional strong man. He left the stage at thirty-three, and was told by his friend that he would go to pieces. He then bet his friend that on his fiftieth birthday he would put up with each hand at least 200 pounds. Remembering the bet, seventeen years later, he elevated with the right hand, on a first attempt, 203½ pounds and the same poundage on a second attempt with his left. I have seen him recently and he appears to be a rugged, sinewy, fifty-year-old man instead of a man of seventy-five. Smith's training consisted to a great extent of exercises which built strength in tendons and sinews. Therefore he never attained the muscular size and shapeliness that other great strong men of his time won, men such as Eugene Sandow, Bobby Pandour or Staff Sergeant Moss of the British Army. Smith's training was the same as that of the famous Arthur Saxon—great emphasis being placed only on heavy exercises, designed to build superior strength in the tendons, muscles and ligaments. Although Saxon is revered for his great strength and for his bent pressing ability for which he was most famous, he excelled at every form of strength feat. He cared nothing for his appearance, cared only about being a strong man, the world's strongest man, and besting the records of previous strong men who had demonstrated their strength in cities that Saxon also visited. By not practicing an all-around training program, not concerning himself about his proportions or maintaining a proper posture, he was actually unsightly in many of his photos. He would be even more famous had he believed that shapeliness comes first, as do most of the devotees of heavy physical training. Instead of spending all of his time at very heavy exercises—many supporting feats, which required great strength particularly in the muscular attachments—if he had shown a fraction of the interest displayed by Eugene Sandow in overcoming his muscular deficiencies, he would have been even more famous today.

As mentioned before I have always been fascinated by feats of strength, but most of all I am interested in building better bodies, in helping my pupils attain the ideal proportions. There is logic in Siegmund Klein's slogan, "Train for shape and strength is sure to follow." Shapeliness alone is not enough; a chorus man may be shapely, but if he is not strong he loses any cause for admiration as far as I am concerned. Strong men, like our weight lifting champions of the day, men who are beautifully proportioned, tremendously strong and the possessors of other desirable physical and mental characteristics, are my ideal. Therefore I prefer a training method to bring the three desired results of building better proportions, which of course requires improved muscular development and at the same time greatly increases strength.

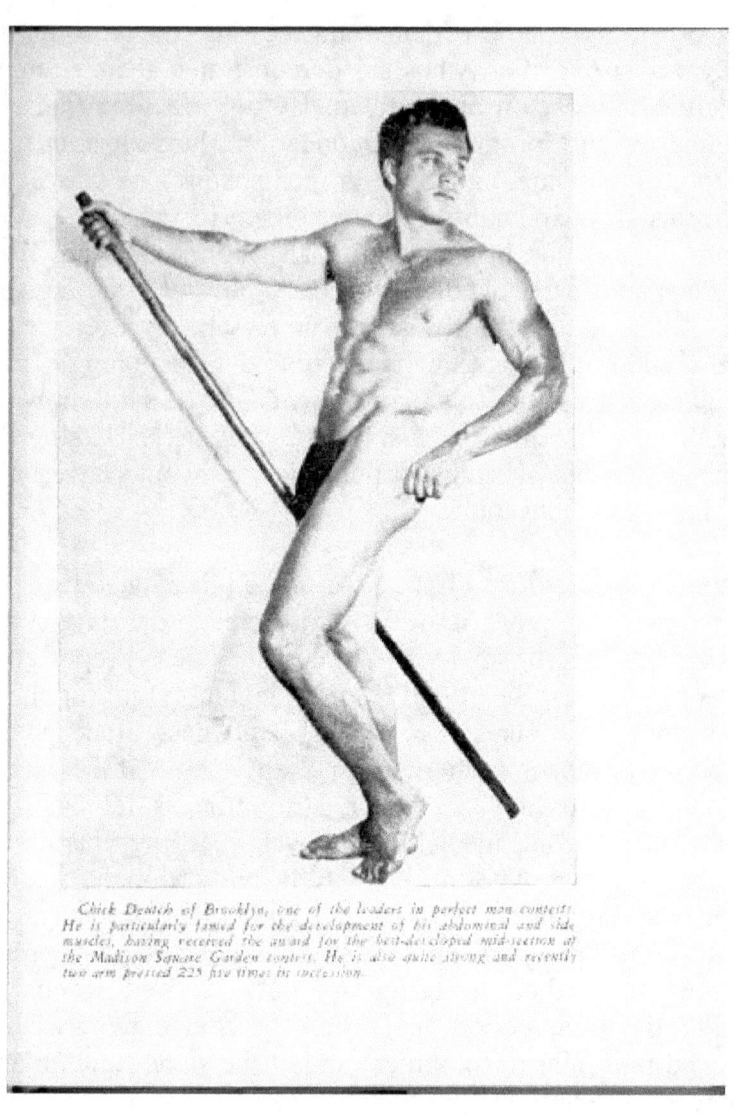

Chick Deutch of Brooklyn, one of the leaders in perfect man contests. He is particularly famed for the development of his abdominal and side muscles, having received the award for the best-developed mid-section at the Madison Square Garden contest. He is also quite strong and recently two arm pressed 225 five times in succession.

In the past it has been generally believed that there are body-building methods and strictly weight lifting systems. So often a young man will write to me stating that he practices only body building, no lifting. Occasionally there is a man who practices only lifting, who attains the heights in

194

the sport of lifting but does not obtain as fine a physique as he should have. When a lifter develops great, strength, but not the best proportions of which his body is capable, it is evident that he has not practiced repetition, progressive exercises to any great extent, nor repetition exercises in his lifts. The members of our own York Bar Bell Club team are good examples of the advantages of all-around training—training for strength, development, perfect or near-perfect proportions, with all the attributes which must be included in the bodies of the champion or near-champion lifters.

Movements devoted to building ligament strength, exercises which are necessary to build a really strong, physically capable body, are not exercises which will alone build the ideal proportions. Ten years ago when the four York bar bell courses were first prepared, they quickly proved to be an ideal training system, one which brought all-around results. The exercises included in these four courses were designed to build every desirable physical quality, particularly great strength, with accompanying muscular size and shape. My own now world-famous twenty weeks' training demonstration to prove the merits of this system made it possible for me to transform my own body, to be much better built and far stronger as proven by my weight lifting ability.

These four York courses are still the ideal physical training method. Not a single word has been changed in these courses in the last ten years. They still contain the best form of physical training, and when a man writes to me or tells me personally when he visits York that he intends to do only body-building exercises, I invariably say, "The best body-building exercises are the repetition weight lifting exercises in York Course No. 3. And it's necessary, too, to lift weights." Others wish to lift and lift and lift—all single heavy attempts. I tell them that this is not enough. They need a more general program, and I still insist and will continue to insist that, whether a man is interested in weight lifting or not, whether he desires to enter competition when some future date is reached, with sufficient proficiency on his own part, whether he is ambitious to be really strong or not, a mixed program of weight lifting and body-building exercises is best.

During my twenty weeks' training I followed the four York courses exactly as they have been sent out to over 100,000 pupils throughout the world—Course No. 1 Monday, Course No. 3 Wednesday, Course No. 2 Thursday, the lifting course Saturday, followed by the practice of some good key exercises. Kindly make up your mind to follow an all-around training program, not merely seeking to build your arms, your body weight or your chest, or to reduce your waistline, but to practice an all-around training program which will bring you the desired physical results of greater strength—strength several times that of the average man, an admiration-creating figure and really sizeable quality muscles, the measurements which are ideal for your type of body and bony framework.

The sort of training method I will constantly write about in the chapters of this book, write about so often that I hope, like dropping water wears away the stone, it will wear away any false ideas or prejudices about physical training that you may have and persuade you to try my "proven to be best" system, is one which primarily increases the size and strength of every one of the four billion muscular fibres which make up your body and greatly strengthen the tendons. As I will constantly reiterate, I admire strength; I am very fond of splendid proportions, but if this strength and shapeliness cannot be converted into athletic ability, I am not satisfied. The famous York champions are not only weight lifting champions but good runners, jumpers both high and broad, they excel at boxing, wrestling, swimming, gymnastics, and make a success at any athletic sport or pastime to which they apply their full interest and efforts.

In the recent Mr. America contest held at Madison Square Garden, as a result of which John Grimek was officially awarded the title by the seven well-known, actually famous judges I presume I should say, as they included Bernarr Macfadden, the living pioneer in physical culture, Colonel Kilpatrick, famous former Yale athlete and president of the Madison Square Garden Corp., Colonel Charles Dieges, great old time athlete, wrestling and lifting champion and for long years one of the leaders in amateur sport, Frank Parker, a famous New York sports writer, Siegmund Klein, famous lifter, bar bell man, instructor, and perfect man in his own right, the possessor of a world- famous physique which couples the strength, proportions and athletic ability about which I am writing, and myself as the seventh judge, there were sixty-one entrants—the very best men in the country. Some of the contestants, notably Frank Stepenek who received the second highest number of points, a New York policeman who possesses considerable athletic ability, Ludwig Schusterich, the lad who before his seventeenth birthday won the title, "Mr. New York," John Gallagher, one of the best lifters in the country, Tony Terlazzo, Elmer Farnham, tri-state Y.M.C.A. champion who was winner of two best-developed man contests in the past, and several others, possessed well-balanced, powerful, symmetrical physiques which bore the marks of all-around training. But too many of the remaining contestants, while possessing on the whole splendid physiques, were not well balanced. It was too evident that they had neglected their legs, their backs, put overemphasis on their abdominal muscles, their arms or their chests. Many of these men had spent their time exercising in front of mirrors, with too few of the movements such as are found in the famous York course

No. 3—the warm up with the half snatch, one arm repetition jerk, one arm stiff legged snatch, two arm rapid press, rapid deep knee bend, holding bell overhead to lower into the squat position, rapid dead weight lift, two arm press behind neck, two arm repetition snatch performed in a variety of manners, two hands repetition jerk, two hands dead hang clean, cleaning without dipping—all exercises which involve the action of all the muscles of the body, instead of building just one group of muscles as do most so-called body-building exercises. They not only develop all the muscles but tie the muscle groups together in co-ordinated action required by these movements. They amplify and strengthen the action of all the internal processes, increase respiration, circulation, perspiration, create appetite, improve digestion, aid elimination, build balance, speed, timing, co-ordination and all desirable physical qualities.

I sincerely hope that my constant pounding upon this idea of all-around training will persuade even those who are "well sold" on weight training that the best results will be had only by following a "proven to be best," all- around training system such as I am offering. I regret to say that some of the men who appeared in that contest, while having great arms, splendid abdominals, finely developed chest muscles, even good legs, were a bit clumsy, did not have proper posture and were not athletic in their general bearing—the result of body-building exercises alone without weight lifting movements or exercises to create the athletic, symmetrical appearance I urge all weight training men to strive for.

Fortunately, the past and present of the greats in the strength world offer many of the type of man I admire most—men with great strength which has been accompanied by superlative beauty of figure. Eugene Sandow—

whom many believe to have been the best-built man of all time, certainly of the past, was also athletic, a hand balancer, wrestler, a tumbler—had as one of his specialties a back somersault with a pair of twenty-five-pound dumbells in his hands. George Hackenschmidt, one of the best-built big men of all time, world's wrestling champion, former cycling champion, the winner of world's lifting titles, and the establisher of world's records, a man who excelled at running, jumping and swimming, was my ideal type. There was Rolandow, famous strong man and great strength athlete who is still living, a man whose feats were almost fantastic. Otto Arco, a small man, with so splendid a physique that he was considered to be the most muscular man in the world, who was and is at the age of sixty-two as this is written a great balancer, a splendid wrestler, as a young man (outweighed over a hundred pounds in many cases) acquitted himself extraordinarily well in European championships which were open to all contestants of every weight; he toured the stage for years and is famed as being one of the greatest balancers the world has ever seen. Fred Rollon was very strong, the possessor of a physique with possibly more muscular definition than that possessed by any other—a human anatomical chart. Bobby Pandour, who would have been more than a close rival of Sandow's if he had received a fraction of the Sandow publicity, had one of the strongest and most symmetrical physiques the world has ever seen and was a fine all-around strength per- former and hand balancer. Antone Matysek, another of the greats of the past, famed for his splendid physique, a man who built himself from the frail beginning of a round- shouldered, flat-chested tailor to great strength as a professional strong man, has these ideal proportions and all- around physical ability we admire so much.

All of the present lifting champions and most of the leading competitors have the ideal all-around development, physical ability and strength. Aside from our own champions, Steve Gob of Petridis A. G., and his teammates, Frank Dorio and John Gallagher, belong in this category. Frank Kay of Chicago, John Terlazzo of German-American, New York, and Dennis Schemanski are only a few of the men of today who possess this much to be desired combination of great strength, muscular size and shape and exceptional athletic ability.

Read this chapter not once but several times, for it contains an all-important message which if heeded will bring you the physical results you crave.

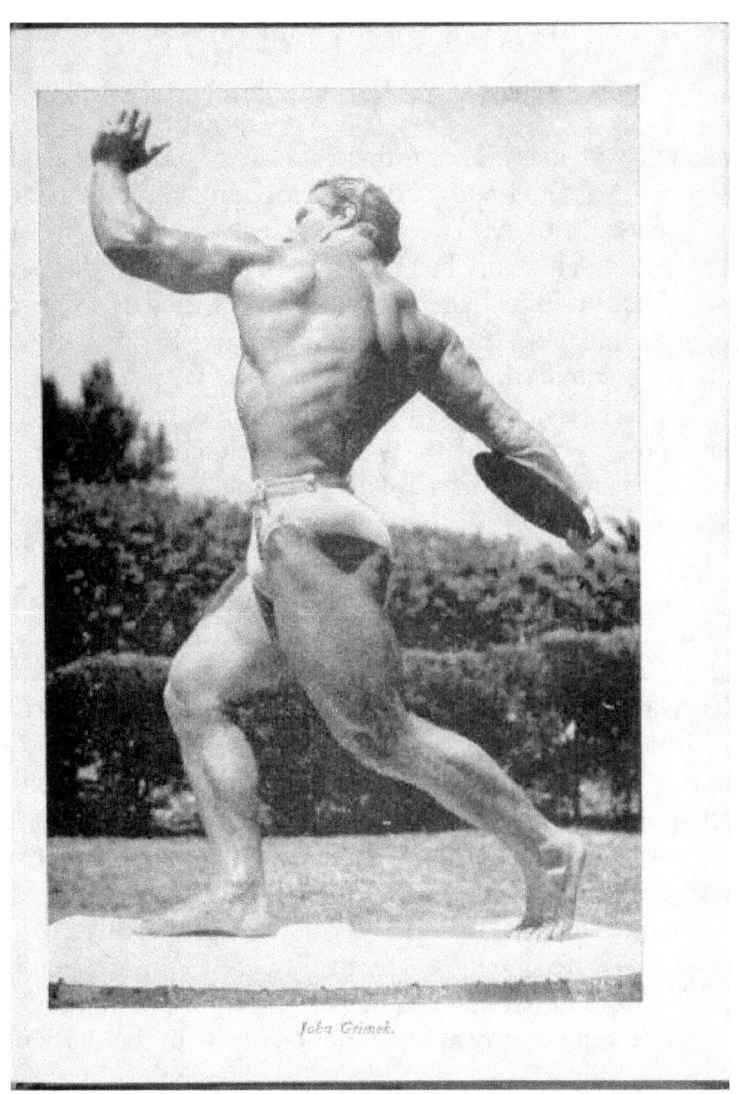

John Grimek.

CHAPTER TWELVE
The Result of Superior Training Methods

The man who has never trained with bar bells when once he launches upon a bodybuilding program should be patient and proceed slowly. He should select a weight in each exercise which can be comfortably handled for five repetitions. A little experimental work will determine the proper poundage. Any normal man should be able to start with fifty pounds in the curl and sixty-five pounds in the two hands press. Some will be able to handle a great deal more; others may find these starting poundages to be too heavy. Be patient; there is plenty of time, and it is better to make haste slowly.

A number of these exercises in the first course will bring into play some long unused muscles, and the first and second day after training you may experience some slight stiffness. But don't be concerned about this. It will wear away in a little while and you will never experience stiffness as you continue with the progressive system. You'll find that your muscles quickly respond to training and in a week or two they will be accustomed to all of the movements. Continue to select the weight for the stated number of repetitions which can be handled correctly and steadily. In the arm exercise press with moderate slowness without bending or twisting, without moving the legs or the trunk to assist in the movements. Perform each movement with the particular muscle group it is designed to develop. Lower the weights slowly, for almost as much benefit can be obtained from this phase of the movement as when the legs or arms are being extended with the resistance of the weight.

Should you be making your start on Monday, all the various exercises will be performed five repetitions. It is wise to work every other day in the beginning, but as this every-other-day system occurs on Sunday every two weeks, many prefer to train a bit differently. Men who are active in some other manner, even working around the house or some form of activity at their work will find three times a week sufficient. This can be Monday, Wednesday and Friday. Thus you have the week end available to do as you like. I prefer to exercise four times a week when I can find time, which is usually before the annual fall strength show held here in York when somehow I manage to take time. This program about which I will write in this and the coming chapter consists of training Monday, Wednesday, Thursday and Saturday. The every-other-day system is 3.5 times per week. I find that three times weekly is hardly sufficient for a man who does nothing in a physical way besides his training. That's why I prefer four days. But ambitious fellows who do not perform any physical work, or at least very light work in earning their livelihood, will train five times a week—moderate with bar bells Monday, moderate with dumbells Tuesday and Thursday, heavier with bar bells Wednesday, rest Friday and Sunday and the limit day of training on Saturday.

These various systems of training all bring good results. The method you are to follow is more easily determined by myself or my helpers here in York, every one of whom is a strength athlete of note. We ask for details, request that you fill out a statistical form telling us your starting measurements, weight, age, physical desires, general health, whether married or single, amount of sleep you obtain, living habits, etc. Then we can more easily prescribe the training system which will bring you best results. Qualified personal instruction and the following of a scientifically arranged and properly outlined system of training are often the difference between splendid success and miserable failure. When you train with the champs, train with us of the

York team, you are sure that you are following the best methods. You have the advantage of personal, qualified instruction.

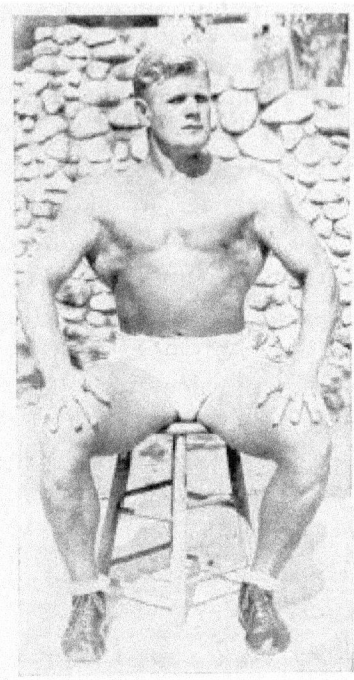

Walter Podolak, at the time he started upon his career as a professional wrestler. Short in stature, he developed a 50-inch chest, one of the largest in proportion to body size of any man in the history of the strength world. He formerly held the world's record in the two hands dead lift at 652 pounds.

To explain our system simply we will assume that you are starting with the every-other-day system. Periods of intensive effort in which regular rest periods are interspersed are an important part of the York training methods. So after your first day of training in which you performed each movement five repetitions, you will rest the next day which is Tuesday. Many young and ambitious strength and development seekers will feel that they can spend their day of rest at chinning, dipping on chairs, swimming or engaging in some other form of physical exercise. If the young man insists on playing baseball and similar games, or following other lines of physical activity such as swimming, wrestling or boxing, this should be done on the training day, either

204

before or after the period of weight training. Nothing in a physical way should be done on the rest day except what is essential in the business of living.

After the day of rest, Wednesday, go through the identical program again, the same poundages and the identical number of repetitions. Rest Thursday and then on Friday you are ready to go ahead. Use the same poundage but practice each movement six repetitions. Rest Saturday and perform six movements again with each exercise on Sunday. Rest Monday, and on Tuesday increase the counts to seven. Rest Wednesday, practice seven movements Thursday, rest Friday, eight movements Saturday, eight the following Monday, nine Wednesday, nine Friday, ten Sunday, ten Tuesday.

If you were sadly out of condition in the beginning, or particularly frail, it might be wise for you on the next training day to reduce the movements to five, as the weight is added to. But most men will have become so accustomed to training in these three weeks that their muscles are already in good condition. The muscles should have responded to training to the extent that all movements can be continued with a minimum of ten counts even with the increase of the poundage. There is little value in performing only five movements, so it is hoped that you have responded to training to an extent which will permit you to go on with the system of training I offer.

Again I must repeat, don't go too fast; if you find that ten movements are too much for you with the increased weight, be satisfied to take your time and drop back one or two movements, working up again with the double progressive system until ten are reached. A minimum of ten movements is required to draw the blood to the working muscles when the most benefit accrues, so ten should be the minimum of movements—preferably twelve or even fifteen —except where the heavy and light system is employed— the three or five times five as will be explained later. In the York courses there is a warm-up exercise and ten other bar bell movements designed to bring into play, with resulting physical benefit, all the major muscle groups of the body. After these ten movements there are seven dumbell exercises. If you are in good condition and ambitious you will find it easy enough to perform these exercises as sort of a rest between the heavier bar bell exercises or after you have completed the bar bell movements.

But if you are not in good condition at the beginning of your training program, if you lack endurance and energy, recuperative ability, until your internal and external strength is improved, until your vital power increases, if you seem too tired after practicing your bar bell exercises, you may find it more advantageous in your particular case to omit the seven dumbell exercises and every third training day practice with dumbells only. On your dumbell night, after you have progressed to Course No. 2 you should practice the dumbell exercises of both Courses No. 1 and No. 2, for fourteen exercises, mostly of a light nature, are not too many.

Men who use the five-day training system may perform only bar bell exercises on Monday, Wednesday and Saturday, and dumbell exercises only on Tuesday and Thursday, or they may practice a full course on the bar bell days. Each man must be his own trainer to a great extent. He knows better than anyone else just how he feels. It is not wise to train hard each training day; a man should work well within himself on some days and husband his nervous energy for the harder, more vigorous once-a-week limit day.

The exercises in York Course No. 2 are the direct opposite of those in Course No. 1. For instance, back hand curl instead of front curl, press behind neck instead of regular press, deep knee bend on toes instead of the flat foot deep knee bend, stiff-legged dead weight lift instead of regular dead lift, etc. So after about four weeks of training it is a good plan to make your start with Course No. 2. You should be ready at this stage of your training to use ten repetitions in all exercises: ten movements with each exercise in Course No. 1 Monday, ten in each movement in Course No. 2 Wednesday, and continue your training alternating in this manner.

Don't be too concerned about the poundages you are handling. Rather be certain that you complete each movement correctly with the muscles that are designed to perform that movement. By this I mean, not using the back in the two arm curl, not jerking, using the legs or bending back in the two arm press. It is best to select a weight in each movement which leaves you comfortably tired at the end of each exercise; not exhausted. While it is true that you must put forth real effort, at least occasionally, you can't do this every night. If you find that eight or nine is your limit on a particular evening, don't force yourself to another count or two on your nerve. Better to stop at eight or nine, building your vital power and reserve energy. The next training period you may have a little more energy and find ten repetitions well within your limit; if not, it's better to reduce the weight a bit so that you can handle the weight for ten movements. Don't increase the weight again until you find it possible to rather easily perform twelve movements; rather fifteen if you wish to make a contest of the particular exercise.

One point of great importance to remember: to build real strength and development you must constantly strive to handle more and more weight. But don't try to go ahead faster than the muscles can properly perform the exercises.

After the second month you should include Course No. 3 in your training program. This is the hardest course of all. Remembering that you benefit in direct proportion to the effort put forth, you will find that faithful following of the weight-lifting exercises in this course will bring the best results of all. Some of the most result-producing exercises in existence are included in this York Course No. 3. It is the combination of the old tried and proven group exercises, with many of these new and original exercises of Courses No. 3 and No. 4 which have resulted in the sensational examples of strength and development from York weight training.

Although you may never have the slightest thought or desire of demonstrating your strength by the lifting of weights you should practice these movements for the results they will bring you. When you have added Course No. 3 to your training program you should practice these three courses on alternate training days: Course No. 1 Monday, for instance, Course No. 3 Wednesday, Course No. 2 Friday. As you progress with your training, you will become bigger and stronger and want to try yourself out at times. I do not recommend that you do this until your muscles are well accustomed to the exercise. But few of us can wait that long; most will try their strength the first day they train with a bar bell. But you will wish to measure your gains; your friends will wish to see what you can lift with your muscles and you will desire to show them. This will give you a lot of fun besides making it possible for you to measure the progress that you are making. It will add interest and variety to your training program. I like the lifting of weights and do not exercise as much as I should. Others prefer to exercise and do not lift as much as they ought to.

It is the judicious balancing of these four courses, these four groups of exercises, which brings the best results in the shortest period of time. When I desire to launch out on a special training program I always train with these four courses just as I am urging you to do.

There is a great deal more interest created when you can have impromptu contests among yourselves. That's the way I like to train. At least one day a week I like to make a fair or a good lifting total, then go back and have pressing, snatching and cleaning contests. These can be arranged on a handicap basis; there is a lot of fun in winning one of these small contests and keeping ahead of the others in your group.

I have been outlining certain definite training principles which have proven themselves in developing scores of thousands of men. There is no longer need for experimental work. The methods of training I am offering you in this and other of my books and in hundreds of magazine articles have proven to be the best methods of training. Just as there are definite, proven-to-be-best principles in machine work, in dentistry, in typewriting, the principles that I am outlining are the only sure way to the acquisition of strength and development. Any form of weight training exercises, if you do not overdo yourself, will bring some favorable consequences, but the best results with the least expenditure of energy will result from following a definite, well-planned course of training exactly as it is written.

I receive scores of letters from men who have my courses who say, "Dear Mr. Hoffman: Will you examine the enclosed course that I am following and see what you think of it?" And a course will be included entirely different from the standard course. Why experiment? It's been done over a period of years and certain exercises and definite training principles have emerged as the best method.

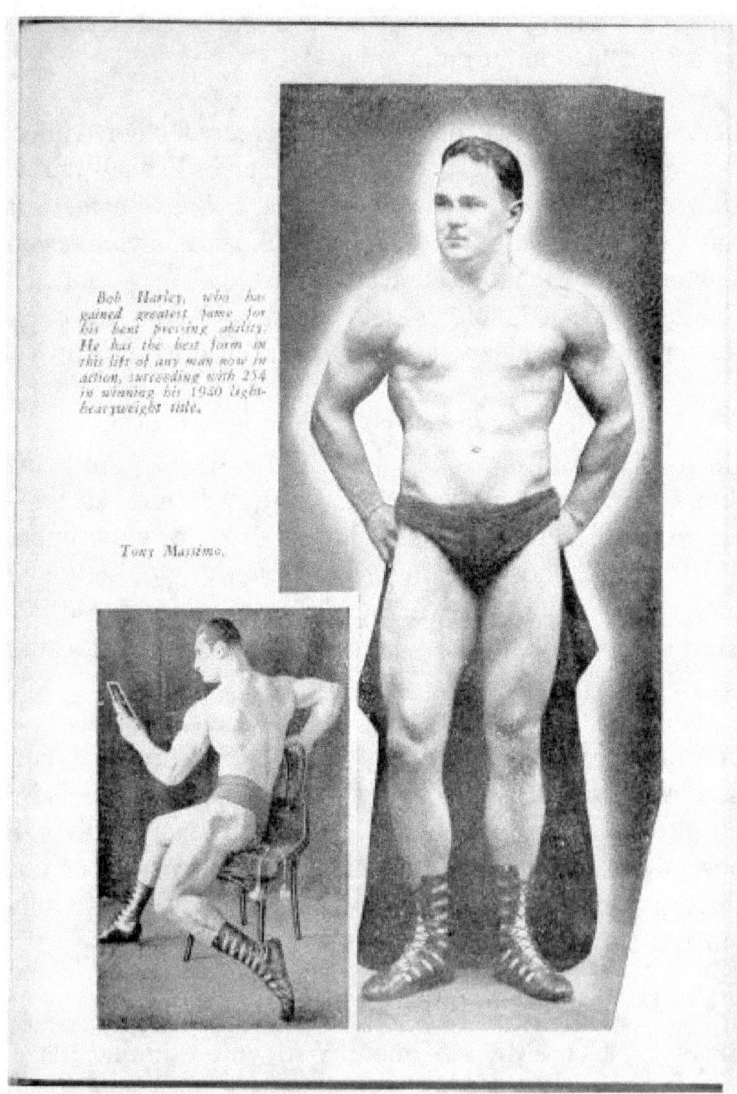

Bob Harley, who has gained greatest fame for his bent pressing ability. He has the best form in this lift of any man now in action, succeeding with 234 in winning his 1940 light-heavyweight title.

Tony Massimo.

A young man visited me recently and asked me why he could not gain weight. I asked him just how he was training.

He said that he was endeavoring to perform thirty deep knee bends, but he could not get past twenty-three. I asked him if he had the York courses. "No," was his reply, "but a friend of mine told me that high repetitions in deep knee bending were the way to gain weight." I asked him if he thought that his friend had had as much experience as we had in body building, and what sort of a physique he had. The young man replied that he had trained very little and was fat and not very strong. And yet he had followed his advice instead of proven advice such as is contained in the York courses and in this book.

"Be warned by my lot, Which I know you will not," are the words of one of Kipling's poems. He hopes that others will be warned by his lot, but in the same breath he admits that he knows they will not. Few humans will heed advice; they must learn, each in turn by his own more or less sad experiences. They are told what they should do, given advice that has proven to be sound, a course of exercises which has proven to be best and still they think they know better. They'll follow their own inclinations or those of some inexperienced friend. They think that their own case is different and with their own ideas of physical training, by some happy accident, some waving of a magic wand, they will be transformed into the man they would like to be.

Of the many visitors who come here to York, many wish to talk over their training problems with me. One young man who came recently had gained fifteen pounds, but only weighed 165 at a height of six feet. He knew how to get stronger, he told me, but it was bulk he wanted, weight and muscular size. He said he knew that the lifting of weights would make him much stronger, but someone had told him that lifting weights would make his muscles so hard that they would not grow. I told him to look around the gymnasium at Dick Bachtell, Wally Zagurski, Tony

211

Terlazzo, Johnny Terpak, John Grimek, Steve Stanko, John Davis and others, weight lifting champions all. I asked him if he would like to be built like any of them. He replied that indeed he would, that he would give anything he had in the world to be built like these champions.

I said, "Then why don't you train like they do?" That sort of floored him for a while. He had not thought of it in that way. Envying these York champions, hoping to be like them, yet he was not following the exercises in the York courses, particularly the exercises of Courses No. 3 and No. 4, which would bring him the results he desired. I questioned him at length about his exercises. I found that he was trying to follow the advice of a number of people instead of the advice of just one, as he should have done. He had started with dynamic tension exercises because he believed that it was best to train light in the beginning, until the muscles were partially developed and toughened. I asked him if he had read that in the York course. He admitted that he had not for the York system starts men right off with the bar bell and dumbell weights they can properly handle.

Dick Bachtell demonstrating some of the best standard barbell exercises. 1. The two hands curl. 2. The two hands press.

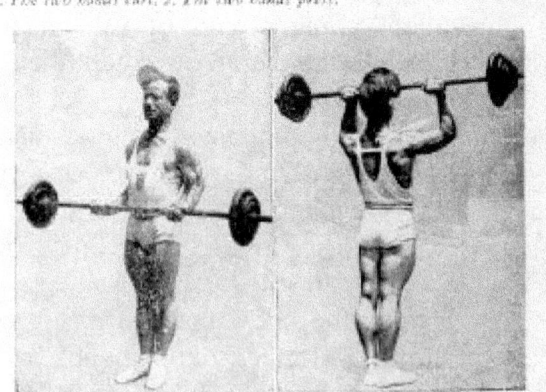

I told him that there were a number of men engaged in the selling of bar bells—one had been a salesman, another is a plumber, another works in a mattress factory, one is a school teacher—who in every case have built nothing to brag about in a physical way. Yet they have their theories —feel that they must differ from our methods, so urge their followers to train a different way. Any man should judge by the results his teacher has obtained. Two other instructors are York pupils; they offer a course basically the same as York. But don't try to follow the advice of more than one man. If you are not sure that I am right, don't follow my advice—train the way a friend or some other instructor tells you, follow your own inclinations, but if you are satisfied that my record has proven that I know my business, follow my system to the exclusion of all others.

There is a reason for every one of the York principles— a reason for the sequence of the York exercises. In each of the York bar bell and dumbell courses there is a warm-up exercise to get the blood action started a bit faster, to stretch and limber the muscles. Then there are two easy exercises to further prepare the muscles for the harder work to come: the two hands curl practiced in a variety of ways in each course and the two hands press. The third regular exercise is the deep knee bend. It is best to perform this heavy movement while you are fresh. This will leave you breathless; and then comes some form of two hands pull over and breathing exercise. Better results are had when you are breathless and are forced to breathe forcefully. And from this point you go on to other York exercises.

213

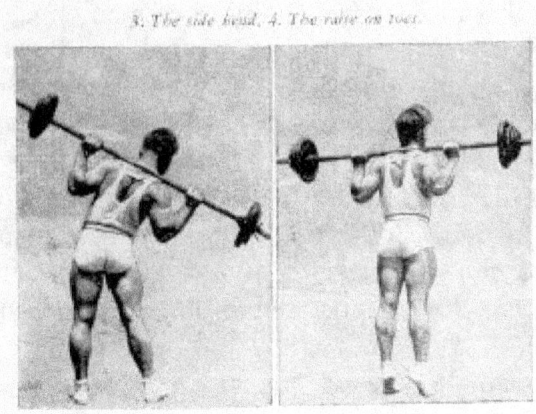

Far better results will be obtained if you follow the courses exactly as they are offered. They permit slight variation, that is, some fellows like to follow the four courses on Monday, Friday and Saturday, with Saturday being a combination of Courses No. 3 and No. 4—trying themselves out with single attempts at lifting to make a lifting total and then continuing with exercises of Course No. 3—and to use Thursday as a "tinkering" day, practicing dumbell, iron boot and cable exercises on this particular day. Some like to have two tinkering days, Tuesday and Thursday, to practice the many good exercises which are not included on the heavier days.

The best results are had with a program consisting of a great many exercises, heavy work and light exercises to build all the muscles, to strengthen the ligaments and tendons, to build endurance, nerve force, to benefit every part of the body. I prefer exercise Monday and Thursday, lifting Wednesday and Saturday, except for the competing weight lifter who must lift weights a great deal more. I prefer to practice bar bell, dumbell, iron boot and cable exercises on the exercise days, and lift and lift and lift on the lifting days. The practice of a great many repetition exercises with

214

substantial poundages on these lifting days will build a real man.

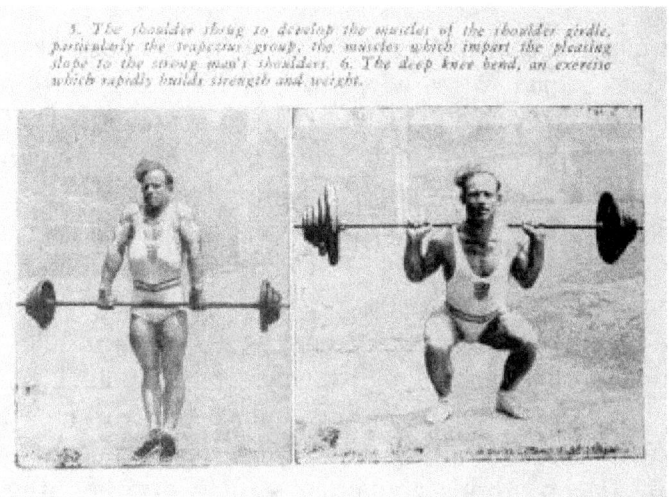

5. The shoulder shrug to develop the muscles of the shoulder girdle, particularly the trapezius group, the muscles which impart the pleasing slope to the strong man's shoulders. 6. The deep knee bend, an exercise which rapidly builds strength and weight.

Regardless of your physical desires, to gain weight, to lose weight, to be a better lifter, this all-around training system will bring you best results. Following such a training program with the observance of other proven York principles will build for you more than your share of strength and development.

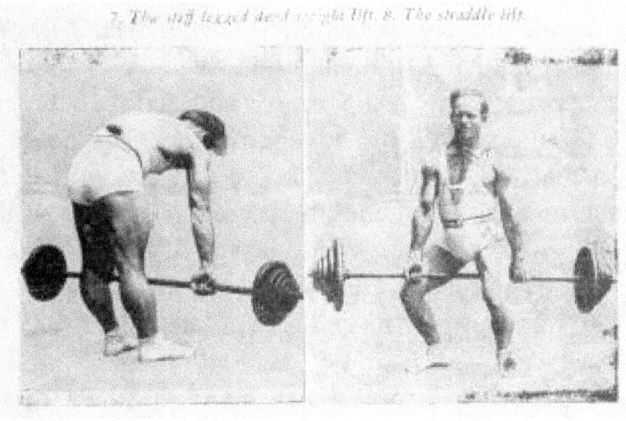

7. The stiff legged dead weight lift. 8. The straddle lift.

CHAPTER THIRTEEN
Additional Successful Training Principles

Irregular training is one of the first of the York principles that has helped so many to success. Your muscles quickly become accustomed to the work they are asked to do. That's why light methods which bring results in the beginning, even during the first seven training days, soon cease to make progress possible. This is because the muscles quickly become accustomed to them, and there is no definite system of progression. If you start out with five- pound dumbells and never increase the poundages, your muscles will become just strong enough to handle that poundage; they will grow only enough to consummate the work demanded of them. You seldom see a pick and shovel laborer who is strong. He performs about the same work day after day, year after year. His muscles become tough enough to continue that particular form of work and never become very strong or well developed. Mail carriers, delivery men, tennis players, Marathon runners, carpenters, or even bricklayers have only average strength; a certain form of endurance is built so that the muscles can continue to do the work asked of them —the workman to work his seven or eight hours, the tennis player to play his five sets, the distance runner to cover as much as the twenty-six miles and some yards of the full Marathon distance. The muscles of these men become just strong enough to do the work asked of them and then the advancing years cut down their ability so that they can no longer do this amount of work. They have no surplus. If they had enough strength, such as the bar bell man, they could lose a part of this strength and still be vastly stronger than average men, and able to continue to do a day's work without great fatigue.

216

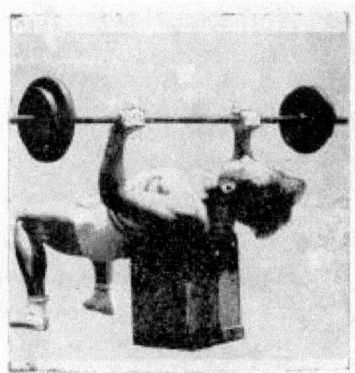

9. The press on box. In this brief course are contained the essentials of an excellent barbell course, which will develop and strengthen all the muscles. To these movements could be added the "wrestler bridge" exercise to develop the neck, the abdominal raise to develop the muscles of the abdomen, and some quicker movements such as the "straddle hop" or the two hands repetition snatch and you would have a single barbell course as good as any.

Something must be done to jolt the muscles out of their regular routine. Therefore after the first proven principle, progressive training, irregular training has its work to do. I popularized this principle of training because it is a training method that I used during a score of years of intensive and successful athletics. I also observed that the strongest men were foremen or bosses of some sort who seldom used their muscles, but occasionally would lend a hand at lifting, moving heavy objects, or unloading heavy material. After that they had plenty of time to rest, usually of days' duration, during which their muscles would be built up and be ready for additional severe demands made upon them some time in the future.

So many of the old time strong men were butchers. Swoboda, Turck, and Steinbach of Vienna held in turn the world's record in the two hands continental jerk. The strongest man was considered to be he who put the most weight overhead. The world is a big place and these Viennese butchers led the world for generations. There must be some reason for it, I thought. Old time butchers would work very hard on their butchering days, using crude and simple old time methods in Europe. They would literally wrestle a large steer, huge hog, kill it, string it up and later carry it in pieces or halves to the refrigerator. After this day of very hard work they would have some days of easy work in their stores or out on their routes with a light wagon. From Turck who first jerked 365 pounds overhead to Swoboda who jerked 440 after it was lifted to his shoulders, the butchers lead the strength parade.

There were old time sailing men such as John Y. Smith who had great power. These old time sailing men would work desperately hard for days at a time in rough weather. This would be followed by days of almost nothing to do, certainly nothing very vigorous. Other strong men worked on beer delivery wagons; they would handle the heavy barrels and kegs on delivery day and have days of rest in between. Stevedores became powerful men. They worked long hours when a ship was in. Steve Gob, one of the most powerful men of his weight in the entire world, a man who pressed 270 pounds officially, who totalled 835 officially, has done considerable work as a stevedore. At times he worked intensively for thirty hours or more, at one time earning $62.00 in continuous work. Then there are long waits between ships. This type of very hard work, followed by long rest periods, had built strong men, while those men who were continually at it built only a form of endurance. Usually they were thin, with corded, stringy muscles and only fair strength.

A study of these results proved one thing: that great demands must be made upon the muscles at times. This we do on the York heavy or limit day of training—a day, usually once a week, in which the ambitious body builder works up to or beyond his best of the past. We train very hard on this day at the York Bar Bell gym. Strangely there is an exhilaration to training in this intensive manner. More glycogen is released by this hard training than is required; there is a surplus which accounts for the great feeling of strength, energy and well being that advanced bar bell men feel on this hard day of training.

It is not possible to train to the limit always, in spite of the rest period which is sandwiched between the training days. More than a single day of rest is required. That's why we usually do not train as severely on Monday as on other days as it is the first training day following the heavy Saturday training. With my preferred training system this is a lighter day, one of the exercise days. Variety is possible during these lighter training days. It can consist of selecting the amount of weight which can be handled ten repetitions. One day of the week it is desirable to select a weight which can be used fifteen times; at other times it is wise to follow the York heavy and light system, or the three times five or the five times five system of training.

Irregular training has proven to be one of the main roads to your physical desires. Kindly remember that your muscles quickly become accustomed to a steady routine with about the same resistance always or even with gradual increases. You must jolt these muscles out of their familiar rut and this is done with irregular training.

In many years of my own training and in coaching thousands of ambitious bar bell men, this system of irregular training has proven to be best. Once a week the athlete should work up to or beyond his limit. That is the night or the afternoon when you break your own records, handle poundages you never lifted before, or exceed the repetitions you have ever made with a certain poundage. The other training days you work out rather moderately. On the first of these, Monday, you could exercise about eighty per cent of your limit, and two days later about ninety per cent of your limit.

Between these heavy days you can, if it suits your ambitions and the time available, have dumbell days, or you can include these with the heavier days, as a partial rest between more vigorous movements or as additional exercises after the harder bar bell exercises. The moderate dumbell days will develop your muscles from many different angles, make them more shapely and stronger. They will tone the muscles and prepare them for the harder days to come. In the dumbell movements you will find that it is at times possible to handle heavy bells and in other exercises from ten- to fifteen-pound dumbells is sufficient. The five-day training system which I employed so successfully during my famous twenty weeks of training, the system with which I established a world's record in physical gains, gains which were more rapid than had ever been officially attained before, is one that I had used during my entire athletic career. In my athletic endeavors, with this system, at the age of sixteen I won my first national championship in open senior competition. During this period of my training, each Saturday I would have races or time trials in training. This of course was my limit day. Two other days I trained quite hard, and two days I took things easy striving for better form and better muscular co-ordination.

This system of training will work well for you if you are one of those ambitious fellows who wish to gain the limit in strength and development. If you are one of the "keep fit" enthusiasts, one fairly hard bar bell day will be sufficient, and two other moderate training days per week. In fact if you are willing to work hard two days a week, you will not only manage to maintain your physique but improve it somewhat. We must remember though that a definite amount of work is necessary to make real gains. I often say that two training periods a week permit you to hold your own, to maintain your physique, three days permit you to gain slowly, but four days of training, at least, permit much more rapid gains.

Concerning repetitions—there are some men who have managed to gain with rather high repetition in some exercises—deep knee bending for instance. I consider ten sufficient in this movement with a heavy weight. Fifteen may not be too many with a more moderate weight and if a very heavy weight is employed I prefer the heavy and light system or a series of bends consisting of five movements each. But there are some like the young man I mentioned who try to reach thirty. A weight must be light to begin or one would never get to thirty. While it is light, little results are obtained in strength and development. Some endurance is created, but usually so many movements leave a man shaken, tired, with "rubber legs," so that he is reluctant to train another day. We have worked out a system of training which does not make great demands upon your nervous energy; rather it builds up these internal qualities so that you have them when they are needed.

Except in some easy movements such as rise on toes, shoulder shrug, the straddle hop, the pull over breathing exercise and similar dumbell movements at which up to twenty counts are permissible, fifteen should be the maximum number of movements. If you want to specialize on a movement, practice it three times ten, or five times ten if you are especially anxious to build that particular part. This way you can use sufficient weight to build muscular power and shapeliness of the muscles. Occasionally there is a superman like Weldon Bullock, the first seventeen-year-old boy in the history of the world to successfully clean and jerk 300 pounds, or like Louis Abele who has made the sensational lifting total of 940, who can perform more heavy deep knee bends. But these men are the exception, who merely prove that the average man should not attempt what they do. Abele has tremendous stores of vital energy; he will sleep ten and even twelve hours, after a hard workout, soundly and well. But these men take several breaths between each bend when the going gets hard so their apparently high repetitions in the deep knee bend are really a series of strength feats. Far better to be satisfied with the weight that you can handle from ten to fifteen movements.

Even ten movements start out easily enough for the first five or six; they become really hard at eight or nine, so that the last one or two are very difficult to perform and are done with a great expenditure of nerve force. This is good for you at times, but not more than once a week. It will cause exhaustion for some rather than rapid progression. Yet it is necessary that heavy weights be used to strengthen muscles, tendons and ligaments, to build the maximum of muscular strength and development, so this is why the York heavy and light system was offered to the strength and development seeking public. It is an exclusive York principle, a copyrighted feature of our courses and one that can be used with bar bell training, weight lifting exercises, dumbell exercises or cable training.

We must remember that at least ten movements are required to bring the blood to the working muscle. Tissue must be broken down, demands must be made, oxygen and, later, more solid food must be required by the working muscle before the blood comes to its rescue. To combine this physiological fact with the need at times to handle very heavy poundages, we need the heavy and light system. With this method a weight is selected which permits seven or eight movements. Almost immediately some of the weight is removed, ten to twenty per cent, and the same movement is performed with this lesser weight for seven to eight counts. We try to reach fifteen in all with this system.

You will find that the second series even with a lesser weight is as hard or harder than the first series.

There is another way to practice this heavy and light system. Using a really heavy weight, one that will permit only three to five exercises, continue until the aggregate number of movements reaches fifteen. This would be three times five or five times three. The heavy and light system is normally practiced but once per week although a host of men have received good results by practicing it every training day. Added strength, development and weight are the usual result of handling these heavy poundages. It is a good way to exercise when you are tired and lack pep.

Many men have had good success by practicing one day only those movements for the upper body and another day only those for the lower. In the York courses the exercises are arranged so that they will be as time saving and as easy as possible while still bringing the desired results. Usually an upper body movement is alternated with one for the mid-section or the lower body. Tony Terlazzo, in particular, has trained with only upper body movements one day and only lower body movements another day. The theory of course is that the major portion of the body's blood will be kept in the part of the body in which the muscles are involved and that better all-around results will be had. The chief objection to this system is the very fatiguing effect it has upon the muscles so that longer and more frequent rest periods with a greater expenditure of time are required to consummate the training program.

It is necessary in order to obtain all-around benefit in strength and development to include in the training program exercises which come under the classifications of paragraphs 1, 2, 3, 4 and 5.

1.   Exercises for building muscles and strength. Exercises to develop the ligaments, cartilages, tendons, and even add to the size and thickness of the bones.

2.   Exercises to build vital force, strengthen the internal organs, improve the process of elimination, improve circulation, develop the endurance of the lungs which is commonly called wind.

3.   Exercises to increase speed, prevent possible slowness, stiffness or sluggishness which might be the result of following too many slow exercises in a training program.

4.   Stretching exercises—those which make the body more supple, flexible, and keep it constantly youthful.

5.   Exercises which develop timing or co-ordination, which develop control and command of the muscles, balance and exactness in all movements.

A variety of good result-producing exercises and routines of exercise are possible while following the proven York principles of training. There is a definite course to fit your particular condition; therefore you will progress best and succeed most if you have qualified personal instruction. Lacking this, the next best form of training for the majority of physical aims is to follow the four York courses exactly as they are offered: exercise Monday and Thursday, lifting and lifting motion exercises Wednesday and Saturday. You'll obtain your physical goal if you follow the advice offered in this volume to the exclusion of any and all others.